Differential Diagnosis in Obstetric and Gynecologic Ultrasound

Second Edition

R A L Bisset
MBBS, FRCR, MHSM
Consultant Radiologist, North Manchester General Hospital and Formerly Booth Hall Children's Hospital, Manchester, UK

A N Khan
MBBS, FRCP (Edin), MRCS, DMRD, FRCR, MHSM
Consultant Radiologist, North Manchester General Hospital, Lecturer in Diagnostic Radiology, Faculty of Medicine, University of Manchester, UK

N B Thomas
BSc, MBBS, MRCS, LRCP, FRCR, MHSM
Consultant Radiologist in charge of Obstetric Ultrasound and Echocardiography, North Manchester General Hospital, Manchester, UK, Honorary Professor, Salford University

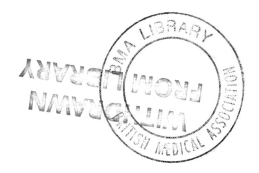

SAUNDERS

Saunders
An imprint of Elsevier Science Limited

First edition 1996

ISBN 0 7020 2681 6

British Library Cataloguing in Publication Data
A catalogue record for this book is available from the British Library

Library of Congress Cataloging in Publication Data
A catalog record for this book is available from the Library of Congress

Drug nomenclature

Directive 92/27/EEC requires use of the Recommended International Non-
proprietary Name (rINN) for medicinal substances. In most cases the British
Approved Name (BAN) and rINN are identical but where they differ the rINN
has been used with the old BAN in parentheses.

There are two important exceptions: adrenaline and noradrenaline, where the
BAN is used first followed by the new rINNS (epinephrine and norepinephrine)
in parentheses.

Drug dosages

Medical knowledge is constantly changing. As new information becomes available,
changes in treatment, procedures, equipment and the use of drugs become
necessary. The editors and the publishers have taken care to ensure that the
information given in this text is accurate and up to date. However, readers are
strongly advised to confirm that the information, especially with regard to drug
usage, complies with the latest legislation and standards of practice.

ELSEVIER SCIENCE your source for books,
journals and multimedia
in the health sciences

www.elsevierhealth.com

The
publisher's
policy is to use
**paper manufactured
from sustainable forests**

Typeset by RDC Tech Group (M) Sdn Bhd
Printed in China by RDC Group Ltd

Differential Diagnosis in
Obstetric and Gynecologic Ultrasound

Commissioning Editor: Michael J Houston
Project Development Manager: Sheila Black
Project Manager: Hilary Hewitt/Camilla Rockwood
Designer: Sarah Russell

Contents

Part 1 Obstetrics

Part 2   Gynecology

Preface to the First Edition

The rapid expansion of medical knowledge has resulted in the production of increasingly large textbooks in every subject. While every department of ultrasonography should have standard works that can be used both for reference and teaching, there is an increasing need for smaller more affordable works. These have the advantage that they can be easily read and annotated with additional information. The absence of images in a textbook of medical imaging is always a disadvantage but does allow the production of a small compact handbook providing a great deal of diagnostic information. This handbook is intended to be just such a text. It has been produced in the same manner as our handbook *Differential Diagnosis in Abdominal Ultrasonography*, by the combination of all our notes taken from lectures, journals, textbooks and practical experience. These have been coauthored by our colleague Dr N.B. Thomas, Consultant Radiologist in charge of Obstetric Ultrasonography at the North Manchester General Hospital. As in our last handbook, the gamut approach to differential diagnosis has been used as it is only by considering every possible diagnosis in a clinical situation that diagnoses can be clinically excluded and a logical choice made.

1996

Preface to the Second Edition

Despite the use of magnetic resonance imaging as a research tool in early pregnancy, ultrasonography remains the modality of choice for antenatal imaging. It is safe, inexpensive and non-invasive. Safety allows repeated use to assess fetal growth whilst image quality allows accurate diagnosis of a large number of structural anomalies. It is the breadth of anomalies that may be demonstrated, the need for early diagnosis and importance of accuracy that make antenatal sonography so challenging. As our understanding of antenatal sonography grows there is an increasing need for short easy reference works that provide a distillation of the major features and complement the larger more comprehensive textbooks.

2002

Introduction

The growth and development of a human baby from a single cell is a long and complex process. There are over 4500 separate structures in the human body and over 90% of these have begun to form by 10 weeks of gestation when the fetus is only 3 cm long. Such a complex process must occasionally fail, and approximately 15% of recognized pregnancies abort spontaneously, the majority in the first 12 weeks; 2.7% of newborn babies have a recognizable congenital malformation of some kind, and normal anatomical variants such as accessory renal arteries occur far more frequently.

Defects in fetal anatomy may be intrinsic or extrinsic in origin. Chromosomal abnormalities may be detected in 1 in 200 babies and are considerably more common in cases of spontaneous abortion. Placental insufficiency may affect a normally formed fetus. Ultrasound provides a direct means of assessing the fetus. The use of ultrasound scanning to assess fetal viability, age, growth, wellbeing, malformations and placental site is now widely established. The number of diseases detected antenatally by ultra-sonography increases almost daily. Ultrasonography provides an image from which the structural development of the fetus can be assessed. Conditions that cause structural changes may thus be identified. These changes, however, may be subtle and difficult to identify, even in late pregnancy. Different diseases with vastly different prognoses may give rise to similar appearances, causing diagnostic confusion, and many congenital diseases remain impossible to diagnose in utero at present. The ultrasonographer examining the fetus may thus be faced with a diagnostic dilemma. Is a fetus normal or is an abnormality present? Could the apparent abnormality be caused by an artifact or anatomical variant. Does the abnormality carry a poor prognosis or will the child have a normal life expectancy and develop-ment? Should other investigations such as amniocentesis be performed, or is there a need for intervention in utero?

To deal with these questions requires a logical analysis of the sono-graphic findings in conjunction with other clinical and laboratory data. The gamut approach to differential diagnosis, so successful in other aspects of diagnostic imaging, can prove very helpful in this situation.

This book is aimed at both those in training in ultrasound and those with more experience. It is not supposed to replace the larger standard texts or current literature, which are essential reading to those working in obstetric or gynecological ultrasound. Many fetal abnormalities are uncommon and will require careful antenatal assessment for correct management, both antenatally and postnatally. Tertiary referral depends on the abnormality in question and is not necessary for minor abnormalities but is appropriate with major anomalies or when soft markers for chromosomal anomaly are seen.

In the gamuts bold type has been used to indicate common abnormalities.

Acronyms and Abbreviations

AA	Aortic arch
ABS	Amniotic band syndrome
AC	Abdominal circumference
ACC	Agenesis of corpus callosum
AF	Amniotic fluid
AFI	Amniotic fluid index
AFP	α-fetoprotein
AP	Anteroposterior
ASD	Atrial septal defect
ATD	Asphyxiating thoracic dystrophy
AV	Atrioventricular
AVM	Arteriovenous malformation
BD	Bipolar diameter
BPD	Biparietal diameter
CFD	Color Flow Doppler
CH	Cystic hygroma
CHD	Congenital heart disease
CMV	Cytomegalovirus
CNS	Central nervous system
CPC	Choroid plexus cysts
CPL	Cystic periventricular leukomalacia
CPVA	Common pulmonary vein atresia
CRL	Crown–rump length
CVS	Cardiovascular system; chorionic villus sampling
3D	Three-dimensional
DA	Diamniotic
DC	Dichorionic
DES	Diethylstilbestrol
DIC	Disseminated intravascular coagulopathy
DWM	Dandy–Walker malformation
EP	Ectopic pregnancy

FH	Fetal hydrops
FL	Femoral length
G6PD	Glucose-6-phosphate dehydrogenase
GIT	Gastrointestinal tract
GS	Gestational sac
HC	Head circumference
hCG	Human chorionic gonadotrophin
ICU	Intensive care unit
ID	Intraocular distance
IUCD	Intrauterine contraceptive device
IUGR	Intrauterine growth retardation
IUP	Intrauterine pregnancy
IVC	Inferior vena cava
IVF	In vitro fertilization
LBWC	Limb-body wall complex
LMP	Last menstrual period
LV	Left ventricle
MA	Monoamniotic
MA	Menstrual age
MC	Monochorionic
MMIHS	Megacystis-microcolon-intestinal hypoperistalsis syndrome
MOM	Multiples of median value
MOPH	Microophthalmia
MSAFP	Maternal serum Alpha-fetoprotein
OD	Ocular diameter
OFD	Occipitofrontal diameter
OH	Oligohydramnios
PA	Pulmonary artery
PC	Pentalogy of Cantrell
PDA	Patent ductus arteriosus
PE	Pleural effusion
PH	Polyhydramnios
PID	Pelvic inflammatory disease
PMP	Premaxillary protrusion
PS	Pterygium syndrome; pulmonary stenosis
PUBS	Percutaneous umbilical blood sampling
PUJ	Pelviureteric junction
PV	Per vaginum; pulmonary vein
RDS	Respiratory distress syndrome
Rh	Rhesus
RSV	Respiratory syncitial virus
RV	Right ventricle

SCT	Sacrococcygeal teratoma
S:D	Systolic:diastolic
SLE	Systemic lupus erythematosus
SUA	Single umbilical artery
SVT	Supraventricular tachycardia
SWS	Sturge–Weber syndrome
TA	Truncus arteriosus
TGA	Transposition of the great vessels
TOF	Tracheoesophageal fistula
TORCH	Toxoplasmosis, other agents, rubella, cytomegalovirus, herpes simplex infections
TTTS	Twin-twin transfusion syndrome
TVS	Transvaginal sonography
US	Ultrasound
UTI	Urinary tract infection
VACTERAL	Association of vertebral, anal, CVS, tracheoesophageal, renal and limb anomalies
VATER	Association of vertebral defects, imperforate anus, tracheoesophageal fistula, and radial and renal dysplasia
VSD	Ventricular septal defect
VUJ	Vesicoureteric junction
YS	Yolk sac

Acknowledgements

The authors are indebted to Paula L Connor DCR, DMU, Anne E Ludlam DCR, DMU and Karen A Mackey, Sonographers at the North Manchester General Hospital, for reading the manuscript and offering constructive criticism of the text.

PART 1

OBSTETRICS

1

Early Pregnancy

Role of Ultrasound in the First Trimester*

- To identify site(s) of pregnancy, e.g. intrauterine, interstitial or ectopic
- To detect early pregnancy failure
- To predict outcome in the presence of a live embryo
- To assess gestational age, uncertain dates or LMP discrepancy
- To determine the number of embryos and assess chorionicity and amnionicity
- To evaluate retained products of conception
- To diagnose gestational trophoblastic disease
- To diagnose some fetal anomalies

With TVS there is improved detection rate of fetal anomaly in the first trimester. However caution is needed in interpreting certain findings in the first trimester such as cystic hygroma, choroid plexus cysts, pyelactasis and echogenic bowel, which may resolve spontaneously. A significant false-negative rate for fetal anomaly has also been recorded in the first trimester of pregnancy.

- To assess associated maternal abnormalities, e.g. ovarian cysts, uterine leiomyomas and retained IUCD
- US-guided chorionic villus sampling
- To assess therapeutic abortion

---

* US should not be used solely as a diagnostic test to confirm the presence of uncomplicated pregnancy.

Further Reading

Levi CC, Dashefsky SM, Holt SC et al (1993) Ultrasound of the first trimester of pregnancy. *Ultrasound Q* 11: 95–123.

Thieme GA & Manco-Johnson ML (2000) A pictorial review of normal obstetric ultrasound. *Ultrasound Q* 15: 106–134.

Predictors of Early Pregnancy Failure

Lack of cardiac activity

Lack of cardiac activity in an embryo of appropriate size indicates death; however, cardiac activity may not be visualized in embryos less than 4 mm in size. A repeat examination should always be considered.

Yolk sac characteristics

The YS functions as a hematopoietic organ and facilitates nutrition transfer in early pregnancy gestation. An abnormal YS is associated with embryonic death and poor pregnancy outcome. Absence of a yolk sac on TVS when GS size is 8 mm or more is said to be 100% sensitive for anembryonic gestation but is not specific and has a positive predictive value of 65%; of the remainder, 22% subsequently develop a viable pregnancy. However the presence or absence of a YS cannot be used to determine if a pregnancy is normal when the GS is smaller than 18 mm. Calcification is associated with a poor prognosis. An abnormal-shaped yolk sac and lack of growth of the yolk sac are further signs of possible pregnancy failure. Unusually large or small YS has been associated with embryonic death. Nevertheless transient abnormalities of YS shape may sometimes occur in normal pregnancies.

Gestational sac features

On TVS, MSD of >18 mm without a yolk sac or >20 mm (mean sac diameter) without an embryo usually indicates pregnancy failure. A distorted GS shape, decidual reaction less than 2 mm, absence of a double decidual reaction and low position of GS within the uterine cavity are other ancillary signs of abnormal pregnancy.

Small sac size: Discordance between MSD and CRL	There is a large range of normal GS size. The peak average difference between MSD and CRL is 14.4 mm at 8 weeks menstrual age, which progressively diminishes to less than 1 mm by 12 weeks menstrual age. Close follow-up is necessary with borderline findings as patients may go on to normal fetal development.
Abnormal amnion	A collapsing amnion, an amnion with irregular margins and when amnion is seen with no visible embryo indicate pregnancy failure. Enlarged amniotic cavity or a yolk sac diameter more than 2 standard deviations above the mean when compared with mean GS diameter is associated with poor outcome.
An 'empty amnion'	Visualization of an amnion but no identifiable embryonic pole is always associated with pregnancy loss.
Fetal bradycardia	The normal heart rate (HR) 6–8 weeks: HR = 111 ± 14/min - 42–45 days. HR = 125 ± 15/min - 46–49 days. HR = 157 ± 13/min - 53–56 days. HR = 80–90/min - 79% loss in the first trimester. HR <70–100% loss in the first trimester. Embryos with HR <85/min during 6–8 weeks do not survive.
	Embryos with slow early HR also have a higher incidence of congenital anomalies as compared to fetuses with normal HR.
Absence of embryo	When no embryo can be identified at 16 mm sac diameter on TVS, 8% subsequently develop live embryos.
Oligohydramnios	OH in the embryonic period indicates a poor outcome.
Low serum hCG	Unusually low serum hCG for the GS size has been described as a predictor of abnormal pregnancy in 65%.

Abnormal CFD

There is no direct contact between embryonic and uterine circulation until the 12th week of gestation. Prior to 12 weeks' gestation sonography reveals no flow through the decidual spiral arteries into the intervillous space, in normal pregnancy. The finding of abnormal flow on CFD in the intervillous spaces and an elevated RI (>0.55) in the spiral arteries are said to be associated with increased prevalence of pregnancy complications, 43% ending in miscarriage.

Subchorionic hematoma

The overall rate of spontaneous miscarriage in a pregnancy associated with a subchorionic hematoma is 9.3%. The loss rate is dependent on the size of the hematoma and maternal age.

Further Reading

Bennall GL, Bromley B, Lieberman E & Benacerraf BR (1996) Subchorionic hemorrhage in first-trimester pregnancies: Prediction of pregnancy outcome with sonography. *Radiology* 200: 803–806.

Doubilet PM, Benson CB & Chow JS (1999) Long-term prognosis of pregnancies complicated by slow embryonic heart rates in early first trimester. *J Ultra Med* 18: 337–341.

Harrow MM (1992) Enlarged amniotic cavity: a new sonographic sign of early embryonic death. *AJR* 158: 359–362.

Jaffe R, Dorgan A & Abramowicz JS (1995) Color Doppler imaging of uteroplacental circulation in the first-trimester: value in predicting pregnancy failure or complication. *AJR* 164: 1255–1258.

Levi CS, Lyons EA, Cheng XH et al (1990) Endovaginal US: demonstration of cardiac activity in embryos less than 5 mm in CRL. *Radiology* 176: 71–74.

Levi SC, Sidney M, Dashefsky SC et al (1993) Ultrasound in the first trimester. *Ultrasound Q* 11: 95–123.

Lindsay DJ, Lovett IS, Lyons EA et al (1992) Yolk sac diameter and shape on endovaginal US: prediction of pregnancy outcome in first trimester. *Radiology* 183: 115–118.

Mara E & Foster GS (2000) Spontaneous regression of a yolk sac associated with embryonic death. *J Ultra Med* 19: 655–656.

McKenna KM, Feldstein VA, Goldstein RB & Filly RA (1995) The empty amnion: a sign of early pregnancy failure. *J Ultrasound Med* 14: 117–121.

Rowling SE, Coleman BC & Langer JE (1997) First-trimester US parameters of failed pregnancy. *Radiology* 203: 211–217.

Stampone C, Nicotra M, Mullinelli C & Cosmi EV (1996) Transvaginal sonography of the yolk sac in normal and abnormal pregnancy. *JCU* 24: 3–9.

First Trimester Anatomy that May Mimic Fetal Anomaly

Fetal rhombencephalon	The rhomboid fossa of the normally developing rhombencephalon can appear as a small (3–4 mm) 'cystic' structure in the posterior aspect of the cranium, between 8 and 10 weeks menstrual age. It should not be confused with an abnormal cystic posterior fossa structure e.g. Dandy–Walker malformation.
Telecephalic and mesencephalic vesicles	Also appear at about 7 weeks.
Physiologic gut herniation	Appears at about 8 weeks and may persist until 12 weeks in 20% of normal fetuses. The umbilical cord may be the site of cysts, varying from 2 to 7 mm, in under 1% of normal pregnancies.

Further Reading

Cyr DR, Mack LA, Nyberg DA et al (1988) Fetal rhombencephalon: normal ultrasound findings. *Radiology* 166: 691–692.

Schmidt W, Yarkoni S, Crelin ES & Hobbins JC (1987) Sonographic visualization of physiologic anterior abdominal wall hernia in the first trimester. *Obstet Gynecol* 69: 911–915.

Skibo LK, Lyons EA & Levi CS (1992) First trimester umbilical cord cysts. *Radiology* 192: 719–722.

Timor-Tritech IE, Monteaqudo A & Warrent WB (1991) Transvaginal ultrasonographic definition of the central nervous system in the first and early second trimester. *Am J Obstet Gynecol* 164: 497–503.

Transient First Trimester Fetal Anomalies

With TVS there is improved detection rate of fetal anomalies in the first trimester. Caution is needed in interpreting certain findings (vide infra).

Increased nuchal translucency
: Nuchal edema in the first trimester is associated with aneuploid states, particularly trisomies 13, 18 and 21. First trimester nuchal edema may be a transient phenomenon and close follow-up is indicated and karyotyping techniques offered if nuchal translucency fail to resolve. The presence of isolated nuchal translucency in the first trimester is associated with a 12.5% prevalence of chromosomal abnormalities and increased risk of spontaneous miscarriage as well as preterm labor. If the fetal karyotype is normal then follow-up scans are recommended; since anomalies such as Noonan syndrome, Joubert syndrome and other non-karyotypic defects may be associated. There is also an association with congenital heart defects.

Nuchal cystic hygroma

Axillary cystic hygroma

Choroid plexus cysts
: Found in 3.6% normal fetuses, investigators are divided on the question of amniocentesis in isolated CPC but most agree that the presence of additional US abnormalities is an indication for amniocentesis. Abnormal karyotype is found in 1–2.4% of fetuses with isolated CPC.

Hydronephrosis	Isolated mild pyelactasis (<3/4 mm) without progressive change is not associated with significant pathology and is found in 3.2% of fetuses. Mild pyelactasis is characterized by a small amount of fluid in the renal pelvis and is affected by maternal hydration. However mild pyelactasis may be a sign of early pathological state. The appropriate threshold for initiating further investigation particularly in the first trimester is controversial but a close watch is essential.
Pericardial effusion	Generally when a fetal pericardial effusion is observed it is along one portion of the ventricle or near an atrioventricular valve, but does not surround the heart. A pericardial effusion surrounding the heart is considered abnormal even when small.
Pleural effusion	
Echogenic bowel	

Further Reading

Babcook CJ, Silvera M, Drake C & Levine D (1998) Effect of maternal hydration on mild fetal pyelactasis. *J Ultra Med* 17: 539–544.

Reynders C, Pauker SP, Benacerraf BR (1997) First trimester isolated nuchal lucency: significance and outcome. *J Ultra Med* 16: 101–105.

Shields LE, Uhrich SB, Easterling TR & Mack LA (1996) Isolated fetal choroid plexus cysts and karyotype analysis: Is it necessary? *J Ultra Med* 15: 389–394.

Intrauterine Fluid Collections that May Mimic a Gestational Sac

A variety of conditions causing fluid collections within the uterine cavity may, in the appropriate clinical setting, mimic a GS. Intrauterine fluid collections lack the double ring margin of an intrauterine pregnancy, and in many of the causes listed below will lack a trophoblastic reaction.

- **Endometrial bleeding**
- **Retained products of conception**
- **Incomplete abortion**
- **Pseudogestational sac of ectopic pregnancy**
- Endometrial carcinoma
- Cervical stenosis/cervical obstruction due to a carcinoma or previous surgery
- Endometritis
- Endometrial arterial aneurysm – this life-threatening condition has been reported only once, on close inspection it was found to be pulsatile on US, while Duplex arterial waveform was detected.

Further Reading

Atri M, Bret PM & Tulandi T (1993) Spontaneous resolution of ectopic pregnancy: initial appearances and evaluation of transvaginal US. *Radiology* 186(1): 83–86.

Jain KA & Grescovich EO (1999) Sonographic spectrum of pelvic vascular malformations in women. *JCU* 27: 523–530.

Empty Gestational Sac

A GS is classed empty when no fetal parts are identified on abdominal scanning in a sac that exceeds 30 mm in diameter or with no YS in a sac that exceeds 20 mm in diameter. Most empty sacs are abnormal in shape.

Normal IUP 5–7 weeks menstrual age	This is less likely with TVS as GS is seen as early as 32 days and is seen in all pregnancies with hCG levels of 1000 mIU/ml.
Blighted ovum	This term applies to arrested development of a fertilized ovum. Most blighted ova are of an abnormal karyotype.
Pseudogestational sac of EP	The double decidual sign is absent in a pseudo-gestational sac.

Positive hCG Without Intrauterine Pregnancy

- Early intrauterine pregnancy <5 weeks gestation
- Recent complete or incomplete abortion
- Ectopic pregnancy
- hCG producing ovarian tumour – germ cell tumour, primary ovarian choriocarcinoma
- Theca lutein cyst associated with pharmacological stimulation with hCG

Ultrasound Features of Early Intrauterine Pregnancy

Gestation sac	A gestation sac is surrounded by an echogenic asymmetrical ring that should be visible at 5 weeks MA on transabdominal US scan whilst on TVS a GS sac is seen at 32 days. A normal sac growth is 0.7–1.75 mm/day (mean = 1.33) from 5–11 weeks. In patients with early pregnancy with a questionable GS a 10 MHz intravaginal probe improves the diagnostic confidence.
Double decidual sac	DDS is useful 4–6 weeks gestational age. It consists of two concentric rings of tissue surrounding a portion of an intrauterine GS. The sign develops as a result of protrusion of the GS into the uterus.
Yolk sac	At 6 weeks MA a YS and amnion should be visible on transabdominal US. On TVS a YS is seen in every pregnancy between 36–40 days and GS between 6–9 mm. YS is seen in 100% normal pregnancies with hCG level 7200 mIU/ml.
Intradecidual sign	When the GS is not sufficiently large to impress, protrude into or deform the uterine central echo-complex and yet the GS is completely embedded within the decidua. This sign precedes the double decidual sign. This sign does not appear to be sensitive or specific in the diagnosis of IUP.
Embryo with heartbeat	Embryo with a heartbeat is expected in all pregnancies >40 days and GS >9 mm on TVS.

Further Reading

Benacerraf BR, Shipp TD & Bromley B (1999) Does the 10-MHz transvaginal transducer improves the diagnostic certainty that an intra-uterine fluid collection is a true gestation sac? *JCU* 27: 374–377.

Dewbury K, Meire H & Cosgrove D (1993) *Ultrasound in Obstetrics & Gynecology.* Edinburgh: Churchill Livingstone.

Laing FC, Brown DL, Price JF et al. (1997) Intradecidual sign: Is it affective in diagnosis of early intrauterine pregnancy? *Radiology* 204: 655–660.

Risk Groups for Ectopic Pregnancy

Ectopic pregnancy rates have increased steadily from 4.5 per 1000 pregnancies in 1970 to 16.8 per 1000 pregnancies in 1987. All females of reproductive age are at risk of EP.

Higher Risk Groups: Ectopic Pregnancy

- Delayed transit of zygote
  Previous tubal pregnancy (10-fold increase)
  Previous tubal surgery
  Previous salpingitis – particularly chlamydia
  Infertility – shared tubal abnormalities with EP

- Infertility
  Ovulation induction
  IVF multiple pregnancy contributory factor
  Gamete intrafollicular transfer – contributory factors include the hydrostatic forces generated during transfer
  Intrauterine contraceptive devices
  History of PID
  Increasing maternal age and parity

Further Reading

Coupet E (1989) Ectopic pregnancy: the surgical epidemic. *J Natl Med Assoc* 81: 567–572.
Zacur HA (1993) Expectant management of ectopic pregnancy. *Radiology* 186: 1112.

Ultrasound Findings in Ectopic Pregnancy

The clinical diagnosis of EP is difficult. The classic triad of pain, vaginal bleeding and a palpable adnexal mass is neither present in all nor specific. The history of a missed period is present in 61% of patients. Ultrasound is helpful in this clinical situation. Correlation of ultrasound finding with serum hCG is essential. A negative ultrasound does not exclude this diagnosis.

Exclusion by demonstrating IUP	US demonstration of IUP makes the concurrence of EP rare, although recent estimates are in the order of 1 in 3000. The incidence is even higher in patients undergoing ovulation induction. In patients undergoing in vitro fertilization the incidence is quoted as 1 in 100.
Direct demonstration of EP	The demonstration of ectopic embryo within an extrauterine mass has been shown in 15–30% on TVS. An adnexal 'ring-like' structure – rounded hypoechoic center surrounded by a thick echogenic ring in the absence of an embryo has been reported in 14–69% and said to be specific to EP. A hemorrhagic ovarian cyst has been termed as the 'great imitator' and may mimic an EP.
Fetal cardiac activity in EP	Fetal cardiac activity when seen on TVS supported by Doppler studies in an extrauterine mass is specific for EP (10% of cases).
Hematosalpinx/complex mass	An adnexal complex mass in the presence of an empty uterus and a positive pregnancy test (hCG) makes the diagnosis of EP highly likely.

Fluid in the cul-de-sac	There are several causes of fluid in the cul-de-sac (see page 416) but when such fluid is seen in conjunction with an adnexal mass and when no IUP can be demonstrated the incidence of EP rises to 70%. If the amount of fluid is moderate to large in association with an adnexal mass, the incidence of EP is even higher and quoted by some to be almost 100%. US is more sensitive than culdiocentesis in detecting hemoperitoneum. The presence of echogenic fluid, which correlates with hemoperitoneum, is highly suggestive of EP especially when a large quantity of echogenic fluid is detected in the presence of an adnexal mass.
Pseudogestational sac	This may occur in up to 20% of patients with EP. The 'double decidual sac' sign (DDS) is a reliable discriminator, being present in a true GS. No yolk sac or embryo will be seen in a pseudo GS. The use of TVS has enhanced the early recognition of both IUP and EP – although it does not absolutely exclude EP nor does it confirm IUP.
Quantitative hCG to US diagnosis: serum progesterone	An empty uterus in an at-risk woman in association with a hCG greater than 1800 IU/l is highly suggestive of the presence of EP. Although this level of hCG is highly suggestive of EP but is not diagnostic. It is reasonable to closely follow-up rather than treat early stable cases of ectopic pregnancy.
Other biochemical aids	Progesterone is produced by the corpus luteum during the early second trimester, until the placenta takes over production of progesterone. A serum progesterone of <5 ng/ml is 99.8% predictive of a non-viable pregnancy either EP or IUP. Progesterone levels measuring at least 25 ng/ml excludes 97.5% of EPs. The levels of progesterone are independent of gestational age so that a single test can be diagnostic without the need for serial examinations.

Endometrial thickness 0.5–1.7 cm	Endometrial changes in the form of a decidual cast occur in 50% of patients and may be indistinguishable from IUP. There is no significant difference in endometrial thickness between women with EP and those with spontaneous abortion. A thin endometrium seen on TVS cannot be used to exclude the diagnosis of EP.
Normal US finding	Earlier reports with the use of abdominal sonography found normal US findings in 20% of patients with EP; however, the use of TVS has reduced this figure considerably.
Doppler sonography in EP	High-velocity, low-impedance flow is identified in both IUP and EP. On spectral Doppler luteal flow can be confused with an EP. It is possible to demonstrate placental flow in an adnexal mass separate from ovary and uterus on transvaginal color flow Doppler. A color flow Doppler may show intense arterial flow adjoining a GS as compared with the rest of the uterus.
Spontaneous resolution of EP	The exact incidence of this is difficult to determine but it is now acknowledged that it occurs.
Endometrial three-layer pattern	A well-defined spherical structure forming three hyperechoic layers separated by two hypoechoic layers within the endometrium has been described with EP. But this sign is controversial and has been described in a variety of conditions besides being a normal appearance. The differential diagnosis of the sign includes early IUP, successful implantation in women undergoing in-vitro fertilization. It has also been described with trophoblastic regression: symptomatic pregnant patients, clinically stable, serum levels of hCG levels below a discriminatory zone, who lack US evidence of either EP or IUP and when symptoms and serological evidence of pregnancy resolve spontaneously.

Further Reading

Atri M (1993) Ectopic pregnancy evaluation with endovaginal color Doppler flow imaging. *Radiology* 187 (1): 19–22.

Atri M, Bret PM & Tulandi T (1993) Spontaneous resolution of ectopic pregnancy: initial appearances and evaluation of transvaginal US. *Radiology* 186: 83–86.

Brown DL (1993) Diagnosis of ectopic pregnancy with endovaginal Color Doppler US. *Radiology* 1187(1): 20–22.

Brown DL & Doubilet PM (1994) Transvaginal sonography for diagnosing ectopic pregnancy: positive criteria and performance characteristics. *J Ultrasound Med* 13: 259–266.

Chen PC, Sickler GK, Dubinsky TJ et al (1998) Sonographic detection of echogenic fluid and correlation with culdiocentesis in evaluation of ectopic pregnancy. *AJR* 170: 1299–1302.

Fellorito JS, Taylor RJW, Quadanc-Case C et al (1992) Ectopic pregnancy evaluation with endovaginal color flow imaging. *Radiology* 183: 407–411.

Hertzberg BS, Kliewer MA & Bowie JD (1999) Adnexal ring sign and hemoperitoneum caused by hemorrhagic ovarian cyst: pitfalls in the sonographic diagnosis of ectopic pregnancy. *AJR* 173: 1301–1302.

Levi CS, Lyons EA, Zheng XH et al (1990) Endovaginal US demonstration of cardiac activity in embryos of less than 5.0 mm in crown-rump length. *Radiology* 176: 71.

Mehta TS, Levine D & Beckwith B (1997) Treatment of ectopic pregnancy: Is human chorionic gonadotrophin level of 2000 iu/ml a reasonable threshold? *Radiology* 205: 569–573.

Mehta TS, Levine D & McArdle CR (1999) Lack of endometrial thickness in predicting the presence of an ectopic pregnancy. *J Ultra Med* 18: 117–122.

Molloy D, Deambrosis W, Keeping D et al (1990) Multisited (heterotopic) pregnancy after in vitro fertilization and gamete intrafallopian transfer. *Fertil Steril* 53: 1068.

Nyberg DA, Hughes MP, Mack LA & Wang KY (1991) Extrauterine findings of ectopic pregnancy at transvaginal US: importance of echogenic fluid. *Radiology* 178: 823–826.

Russell S, Filly RA & Damanto N (1993) Sonographic diagnosis of ectopic pregnancy with EV probes; what really has changed? *J Ultrasound Med* 12:145.

Wachsberg RH (1998) Ectopic pregnancy: recent developments and changing concepts. *J Clin Ultrasound* 14: 247–253.

Wachsberg RH (2000) Pitfalls in the sonographic diagnosis of ectopic pregnancy. *Ultrasound Q* 16: 89–96.

Wachsberg RH, Karimi S (1998) Sonographic endometrial three layer pattern in symptomatic first trimester pregnancy: not diagnostic of ectopic pregnancy. *JCU* 26: 199–201.

Differential Diagnosis of Ectopic Pregnancy

- **Any adnexal mass**
- All causes of fluid in the cul-de-sac
- Corpus luteum cysts with/without septa
- Torsion of ovarian cyst/neoplasm
- **Endometriosis**
- **Tubo-ovarian abscess**
- Torsion/degeneration of a fibroid
- Ovarian neoplasm
- Hemorrhagic ovarian cyst
- Uterine leiomyoma
- Hemorrhagic subserosal fibroid
- Appendix abscess
- Diverticular abscess

Further Reading

Hertzberg BS, Kliewer MA & Bowie JD (1999) Adnexal ring sign and hemoperitoneum caused by hemorrhagic ovarian cyst: pitfall in the sonographic diagnosis of ectopic pregnancy. *AJR* 173: 1301–1302.

Parvery HR & Markland N (1993) Pitfalls in transvaginal sonographic diagnoses of ectopic pregnancy. *J Ultrasound Med* 3: 139–144.

Russell SA, Filly RA & Damato N (1993) Sonographic diagnosis of ectopic pregnancy with endovaginal probes: what really has changed? *J Ultrasound Med* 3: 145–151.

Ultrasound Parameters for Measurement of Gestational Age

Approximate age (weeks) Post LMP	
5-6	Gestational sac volume
7-12	Crown-rump length
12-15	BPD, femoral length, head circumference
24	After 24 weeks, individual variation in fetal size and growth render sonographic estimation of fetal age inaccurate. (Foot length may be helpful.)
Gestational sac size	GS can be visualized from 4 weeks on TVS and 5-6 weeks at trans-abdominal US. The sac is usually ovoid, therefore when the sac diameter is calculated an average of AP, transverse and longitudinal diameters is taken. When the sac is round only one measurement is necessary. The measurements are taken from the internal borders - mean sac diameter. Sac volume is calculated as AP × transverse × length × 0.5223.
Crown-rump length	This is the most accurate means of dating a pregnancy and is less likely than the GS measurement to be affected by external factors such as uterine compression by the urinary bladder in early pregnancy. It is affected by fetal flexion as the fetus matures. CRL measurement is not affected by maternal age, height, parity or racial origin. The accuracy of CRL measurement/ gestational age prediction is ±5-7 days.
Biparietal diameter	Once the internal anatomy of the fetus can be clearly identified, standard landmarks can be used to obtain measurements. The fetal BPD diameter is one such measurement and is the most widely used means of assessing gestational age. It is accurate ±5 days.

Femoral length

The femoral length may be measured from 12 weeks. It does not replace the BPD entirely satisfactorily but rather should be used to confirm results from BPD measurements. It is of particular value if the fetal skull lies deep in the pelvis and a good section for BPD estimation cannot be obtained. Any of the long bones of the fetus can be measured, the femur is preferred because it is the longest and easiest to image.

Other Fetal Measurements

Abdominal circumference	This is used: (1) to assess fetal growth; (2) to evaluate any disproportion between head and body size; (3) to evaluate appropriate fetal growth over a period of time.
Head circumference	The head circumference may be measured directly by marking the margins of the skull or indirectly by the formula: Head circumference = (BPD + OFD) × 1.62.
Multiple parameter (BPD, FL, HC, etc)	Averaging the results of multiple parameters is not universally accepted. Proponents state it results in approximately 25% increase in accuracy in predicting gestational age. Their main limiting factor in later pregnancy is the increasing importance of genetic variation and alteration in growth, therefore the measurement cannot accurately predict gestational age after 24 weeks.
Fetal weight	Analysis of fetal weight may be performed using standard fetal measurement (AC, HC, FL, BPD, etc.), either as single parameters (AC) or in combination of up to 4. The use of AC gives accuracy of ±160 g/kg fetal weight. Combining the use of BPD and AC increases accuracy to ±106 g/kg but adding further parameters improves accuracy by no more than 1%. The fetal weight is estimated by measuring the chosen parameters and comparing them with standard charts for weight. Unfortunately, all the formulae tend to overestimate the weight of the low birthweight fetus, although most have an overall accuracy within ±10%. In future 3D ultrasound may give us better estimates.

Fetal foot length

There are limitations to the use of fetal foot length for gestation age assessment particularly in fetuses with growth abnormalities.

Causes of Inaccuracy in Estimating Gestational Age from Menstrual History

- LMP date not accurately known
- Cycle is irregular
- Cycle is not 28 days long
- Bleeding in early pregnancy may mimic a menstrual period
- Contraceptive pill recently used as a form of contraception
- Post delivery breast feeding

Advantages of Ultrasound Estimation of Gestational Age

- Allows accurate planning for an estimated date of delivery.
- Permits appropriate steps to be taken should labor start before 38 weeks or fail to start by 42 weeks, to ensure optimum fetal outcome.
- Is vital for the correct interpretation of screening blood tests such as AFP, hCG level in screening protocols.
- Is essential for the timing of later scans to detect fetal anomalies and is required for the interpretation of most ultrasound fetal parameters, i.e. femoral length, head circumference, etc.
- Is also required for the assessment of fetal growth because the rate of growth depends upon fetal age and the normal range for many of the commonly used fetal parameters increases with age.

Further Reading

Fetal Measurements Working Party (1990) *Clinical Applications of Ultrasound Fetal Measurements*. British Institute of Radiology/British Medical Ultrasound Society, London.

Frank P & Hadlock FP (1990) Sonographic estimation of fetal age and weight. *Radiol Clin North Am* 28: 39–51.

Hadlock FP (1994) *Ultrasonography in Obstetrics and Gynecology*, 3rd edn, pp 129–143. Philadelphia: WB Saunders.

Hadlock FP, Deter RL, Harrist RB & Park SK (1982) Fetal HC: relationship to menstrual age. *AJR* 138: 647–653.

Kurjack A, Crvenkovic G, Salihagic A et al (1993) Assessment of normal early pregnancy by transvaginal color Doppler ultrasonography. *JCU* 21(1): 3–8.

Lee W, Comstock CH, Kirk JS et al (1997) Birth weight prediction by three-dimensional ultrasonographic volumes of the fetal thigh and abdomen. *J Ultra Med* 16: 799–805.

Meirowitz NB, Ananth CV, Smulian JC et al (2000) Foot length in fetuses with abnormal growth. *J Ultra Med* 19: 201–205.

Pinette MG, Pan Y, Pinette SG et al (1999) Estimation of fetal weight: mean value from multiple formulae. *J Ultra Med* 18: 813–817.

Robinson HD & Fleming JEE (1975) A critical evaluation of sonar crown-rump length measurements. *Br J Obstet Gynaecol* 82: 702–710.

Corpus Luteum in Early Pregnancy

The corpus luteum (CL) is identified in the first trimester on TVS in most pregnancies. This physiological structure produces progesterone, which sustains pregnancy until the placenta is formed. At around 7 weeks gestation the functioning CL is no longer necessary because the placenta assumes hormonal function. Consequently it decreases in size during 8–16 weeks gestation and is subsequently maintained passively for the rest of the term of pregnancy.

- Varied US appearances with a mean diameter of 1.9 ± 0.6 cm (range 0.8–5.5 cm)
- Hypoechoic – 34%
- Cystic with thick circumferential wall and anechoic center – 27%
- Cyst with scattered echoes or internal debris – 23%
- Thin-walled simple cyst – 15%
- No CL identified – 2%
- Circumferential flow partial or all CL on Color flow Doppler – 92%
- Flow on pulsed Doppler in 92% with a mean resistive index of 0.49 ± 0.08 (range 0.29–0.91)

Further Reading

Durfee SM & Frates MC (1999) Sonographic spectrum of the corpus luteum in early pregnancy: gray scale, Color and pulsed Doppler. *JCU* 27: 55–59.

The Cervix in Pregnancy

Normal cervix in pregnancy	It is usually difficult to distinguish cervix from the lower uterine segment in the non-gravid state and the first trimester. From mid-trimester onwards the amniotic sac clearly defines the internal os. US has advantages over digital examination; the internal os can be visualized by sonography and hence detect early changes of cervical incompetence and moreover there is a decreased risk of infection and cervical irritation.
Cervical length	Cervical length is the distance between the internal and external os. First trimester cervical length: >5 cm. Cervical length decrease to <34 mm at 28 weeks gestation. There is no difference in the cervical length between the nulliparous or multiparous. In patients with multiple gestation there is significantly shorter cervical length. Normograms have been developed for twins and triplets that help to identify patients at high risk of preterm labor.
Preterm labor	There is an inverse relationship between US cervical length and the risk of preterm labor. Length <25 mm at 24 weeks gestation = 4-fold increased risk of preterm labor. Funneling/ wedging of the internal os with prolapse of fetal membrane is indicative of the onset of preterm labor. Funneling of over 60% of the length of the cervical canal is also associated with preterm labor.
Incompetent cervix	Cervical incompetence is defined as cervical dilatation without uterine contractions. In patients with history of pregnancy loss it is prudent to establish a baseline cervical length measurement before the gestation age when the previous loss occurred with follow-up scans 1–2 weeks depending upon the findings or recent examination or symptoms. TVS com-

bined with transfundal pressure or scanning patient in a standing position can illicit early changes.

Dynamic changing cervix

This dramatic event can be seen during US examination. The cervix show dynamic changes with varying degree of funneling of the internal os associated with vigorous closing and opening of the cervix. These changes occur in the absence of uterine contractions. Although most patients with a spontaneously changing cervix deliver pre-term it is not a sign of imminent delivery and with conservative management delivery may be delayed in some.

Cervical cerclage

Sonographic guidance can be used to assist placement of cervical cerclage as a prophylaxis to preterm labor in cervical incompetence. Following placement of cervical cerclage, measurements of the canal are made from the internal os to the level of cerclage. Shortening of the upper cervical length <1 cm is associated with preterm delivery.

The cervix at term

Several recent studies using US to evaluate the ripeness and inducibility of cervix have been published and a scoring system has been proposed. Parameters such as cervical length, cervical diameter and the appearance of the internal os are scored. Using these indices it has been shown that the presence of funneling and a short cervical length is associated with a shorter duration of induced labor. US has been shown to correlate well with digital examination; however the firmness of the cervix, which is an important sign of the ripeness of the cervix can only be assessed digitally. US technique is useful in patients in whom digital examination is contraindicated such as in patients with premature rupture of membranes and unexplained vaginal bleeding.

False Positive Findings of Incompetent Cervix

- Uterine contraction – differentiated by the observation of a thickened myometrium associated with uterine contractions, palpation of the uterus, placement of tocodynamometer and questioning the patient may disclose the presence of uterine contractions.
- Narrowed lower uterine segment can mimic funneling – clarified by observing the cervix over time.
- Overdistended urinary bladder impression on the lower uterine segment may produce the impression of funneling of the cervix.
- Cystic lesions such as Nabothian cysts and vaginal cyst can mimic a dilated internal os.

Incompetent Cervix: Risk Factors

- DES exposure in utero associated with cervical hypoplasia
- Previous cone biopsy of the cervix
- Prior cervical laceration
- Prior cervical trauma – cauterization, dilatation and curettage, etc.
- Estrogen therapy

Further Reading

Hertzberg BS, Kliewer MA, Farrell TA & DeLong DM (1995) Spontaneously changing gravid uterus: clinical implications and prognostic features. *Radiology* 196: 721–724.

Imseis H, Albert T & Iams J (1997) Identifying twin gestations at low risk for preterm birth with a transvaginal sonographic measurement at 24–26 weeks gestation. *Am J Obstet Gynecol* 177: 1149–1155.

Kushnir O, Izquierdo L, Smith J et al (1995) Transvaginal sonographic measurement of cervical length: evaluation of twin pregnancy. *J Reprod Med* 40: 380–382.

Ludmin J, Abbott J, Wong G et al (1995) Vaginal sonography of the cervix in the management of triplet gestation. *Am J Obstet Gynecol* 172: 407.

Michaels W, Schreiber F, Ager J et al (1991) Ultrasound surveillance of the cervix in twin gestation: management of cervical incompetence. *Obstet Gynecol* 78: 739–749.

Wong G, Levine D (1998) Sonographic assessment of the cervix in pregnancy. *Seminars Ultrasound, CT & MRI* 19: 370–380.

Abortion

There is a 10–25% pregnancy loss rate of all clinically diagnosed pregnancies. The majority of the losses occur before the 7th week gestation usually due to abnormal karyotype of which 52% are trisomies, 20% triploidy and 15% monosomy.

Complete abortion products	There is complete loss of conception with a closed cervix and a thin endometrium on US.
Incomplete spontaneous abortion	There are retained products of conception with continued bleeding associated with a patulous cervix. The retained products may represent placental tissue or fetal tissue. US findings include: gestational sac/fluid collection; GS with a dead fetus; endometrial thickness >5 mm in the majority but thickness may vary from 2–5 mm, in 14% thickness may be 2 mm or less. Complications include endometritis, septicemia, and diffuse intravascular coagulation.
Inevitable abortion	The GS becomes detached from its implantation site within the uterus so that abortion becomes inevitable and abortion usually occurs within a few hours. Presentation is usually with PV bleeding <7 days, persistent painful uterine contractions, a dilated cervix and ruptured membranes. US findings include: a GS low within the uterus; GS surrounded by an anechoic zone of blood and a dilated cervix.
Missed abortion	This usually occurs between 8–14 weeks gestation. There is a dead conceptus within the uterus usually associated with a brownish vaginal discharge with a closed cervix. US features include, no cardiac activity in the embryo of appropriate size, gestation inappropriate for menstrual age, GS >25 mm with no embryo, GS >20 mm without a YS, misshapen GS, debris within the GS, lack of a double decidual sac, a low sac position and a sub-chorionic fluid collection.

Threatened abortion

First trimester PV bleeding associated with a live fetus and closed cervix. The incidence is 20–25% of all clinically apparent pregnancies with a 50% pregnancy loss rate. Fetal viability depends on detection of fetal heart beat and movement. Early fetal bradycardia, relative fetal inactivity and the presence of a large sub-chorionic hematoma are poor prognostic signs.

Fetal Anomalies Detectable on Ultrasound in the First Trimester

Head and neck	**Cystic hygroma**
	Nuchal translucency
	Anencephaly
	Large cranial cysts
	Exencephaly
	Encephalocele
	Acrania
	Choroid plexus cysts
	Dandy-Walker malformation
Spine	Neural tube defects
	Kyphoscoliosis
Ventral	Omphalocele
	Gastroschisis
	Ectopia cordis
	Lateral fold defect
Extremities	Short limb dysplasia
Heart	Atrioventricular canal defect
	Complete heart block
Genitourinary	Hydronephrosis
	Megacystis
	Cystic dysplastic kidneys
Placenta, umbilical cord and yolk sac	Partial mole
	Umbilical cord cysts
	Short cord associated with ventral fold defect
	Large yolk sac
Multiple gestation	Monoamniotic twins
	Twin-twin transfusion syndrome
	Conjoined twins

NB   Most first trimester anomalies are more clearly visualized using TVS. Many serious anomalies may have a normal sonogram in the first trimester of pregnancy – anencephaly becomes obvious after ossification of the calvarium at or after 12 weeks of menstrual age.

Further Reading

Achivon R, Achron A & Yagel S (1993) First trimester for transvaginal sonographic diagnosis of Dandy-Walker malformation. *J Ultrasound Med* 21: 62–64.

Bennett JC, Burlbaw J, Drake CK & Finley BE (1991) Diagnoses of ectopia cordis at 12 weeks gestation using transabdominal ultrasonograph with color flow Doppler. *J Ultrasound Med* 10: 695–696.

Cullen MT, Green J, Whetham J et al (1990) Transvaginal ultrasonographic detection of congenital anomalies in the first trimester. *Am J Obstet Gynecol* 163: 466–476.

Goldstein RD & Filley RA (1988) Prenatal diagnoses of anencephaly: spectrum of sonographic appearances and distinction from the amniotic band syndrome. *AJR* 151: 547–550.

Timor-Tritsch IE, Monteaqudo A & Peisner DB (1992) High frequency transvaginal sonographic examination for the potential malformation assessment of the 9 week to 14 week fetus. *JCU* 20: 231–238.

Van Zalen-Sprock RM, van Vugt JM & van Geijn HP (1995) First and early second trimester diagnosis of anomalies of the central nervous system. *J Ultrasound Med* 14: 603–610.

2

Fetal Wellbeing and Growth

Biophysical Profile

The biophysical profile is a means of assessing fetal wellbeing utilizing five measurable parameters. Each parameter is given a score of 0–10. Ventzileos et al (1983) have added placental grade to the profile, although placental grading is not used in most departments. Low scores are associated with poor outcome. The following parameters are included in the assessment.

Fetal breathing movement

Real time US is used to assess breathing movements. The presence of at least one period of breathing lasting 60 seconds or more in a 30-minute period is considered normal. Hiccup and fetal movements are not counted.

Scoring
2 = 30 seconds sustained breathing/30 minutes
0 = < 30 seconds of sustained breathing/30 minutes.

Fetal movements

Gross movements are recorded over 30 minutes: simultaneous limb and trunk movements are scored as a single event. Three movements over a 30-minute period are considered normal. The fetus is most active 1 hour after the mother has eaten.

Scoring
2 = 3 gross movements/30 minutes
0 = <3 movements/30 minutes.

Fetal tone

Flexion of the trunk with both the upper and lower limbs flexed is considered normal. If fetal extension is not followed rapidly by flexion, or the spine is extended with extended limbs or only partially flexed limbs, then tone is reduced. These fetuses hold their hands 'open.'

Scoring
2 = closed fists, flexed fetus/flexion from extension
0 = neither of above.

Amniotic fluid volume

Amniotic fluid volume is measured in areas free of small parts. OH is present when the largest pocket of fluid is less than 2 cm. A four-quadrant assessment is however usually made; the sum of fluid depths (amniotic fluid index) should be more than 5 cm.

Scoring
2 = pockets of amniotic fluid >1 cm, i.e., normal liquor volume
0 = pockets of amniotic fluid <1 cm, i.e., oligohydramnios.

Non-stress test

The fetal heart rate is continuously monitored with Doppler ultrasound with simultaneous assessment of fetal movement by tachynamometer. Two accelerations of fetal heart rate of at least 15 beats/min above the baseline, associated with fetal movements lasting at least 15 seconds, must be present within a 20 min period for the test to be positive

Scoring
2 = 2 or more accelerations/20 minutes
0 = <2 accelerations.

Nuchal cord compression stress test

External pressure with the ultrasound probe is applied over the nuchal cord for 10 seconds, causing venous occlusion (assessed on color Doppler). The fetal heart rate rises by 20–30 beats/min after the pressure is released, returning to normal by 60 seconds. This response is reduced or absent when the fetus is hypoxic.

Placental grade

Echogenicity and appearance of the maturing placenta have been used to assess placental grading (see p. 88): placental grade does not correlate well with fetal outcome and is therefore not included in the biophysical score in most departments.

Scoring
2 = grade 0, 1 or 2 placenta
1 = indeterminate placenta
0 = grade 3 placenta.

Biophysical profile and steroids

Biophysical fetal profile score decreases by 2–4 points within 48 hours after antenatal steroids administration in one third of the cases. Fetal breathing and the non-stress test are the most common parameters affected. However a borderline low biophysical profile score (4 or 6) in the setting of recently administered steroid is not a prediction of fetal distress and does not affect neonatal outcome.

Doppler waveform abnormalities

Although Doppler waveforms are not included in the scoring system, umbilical cord arterial waveforms appear to be the most accurate predictors of poor neonatal outcome in small-for-gestational-age fetuses. Poor outcome can occur when the biophysical profile and non-stress tests are normal, but the umbilical cord arterial waveforms are abnormal. A systolic: diastolic ratio greater than 4.0 is a predictor of poor neonatal outcome.

Heart Rates in Early Pregnancy

6–8 Gestation Weeks:

Heart rate: 111 ± 14/min – 42–45 days
Heart rate: 125 ± 15/min – 46–49 days
Heart rate: 157 ± 13/min – 53–56 days.

Heart rate 80–90 – 79% loss rate in the first trimester
Heart rate <70 = 100% loss
Embryos with HR 85 beats/min and below during 6–8 weeks do not survive.

Fetal Macrosomia

A macrosomic fetus is defined as weight >4000 grams. Fetal macrosomia is associated with increased perinatal morbidity and mortality. Perinatal mortality increases from 3.5 per 1000 births for infants weighing 2500–3500 grams to 8 per 1000 births for infants weighing >4500 grams. Macrosomic infants are more likely to experience birth trauma such as limb bone fractures, shoulder dystocia and brachial plexus injury. A variety of US methods have been used to estimate fetal weight. There is a wide range of predictive value for fetal weight estimation calculated from BPD, AC and limb measurement. An abnormally thick subcutaneous tissue at the level of the thigh >2 SD above mean is found in 23.7% of macrosomic fetuses. Fetal abdominal subcutaneous tissue thickness varies from 3–18 mm with a mean measurement of 8.4 ± 2.7 mm (standard deviation). The mean tissue thickness differs significantly between normal and macrosomic fetuses (7.00 versus 12.4 mm respectively).

Conditions Associated with an Adverse Outcome in a Structurally and Genetically Normal Infant

Postmaturity

Pregnancy is not usually allowed to progress beyond 42 weeks. Accurate dating in early pregnancy is essential. At postmaturity ultrasound may show oligohydramnios, skin wrinkling. Growth retardation late in pregnancy may also be associated with meconium aspiration.

Prematurity

Delivery prior to term, i.e., before 36–42 weeks.

Growth retardation

Further Reading

Birnholz JC (1990) Ecologic physiology of the fetus: ultrasonography of supply-line deprivation syndromes. *Radiol Clin North Am* 28: 179–188.

Deter RL, Harrist RB: (1993) Assessment of normal fetal growth. In Chervenak FA, Isaacson GC, Campbell S (eds) *Ultrasound in Obstetrics and Gynecology.* Boston, Little Brown & Co, p 361.

Dubinsky T, Lau M, Powell F et al (1997) Predicting poor neonatal outcome: a comparative study of noninvasive antenatal testing methods. *AJR* 168: 827–831.

Frates MC, Benson CB & Doubilet PM (1993) Pregnancy outcome after a first trimester sonogram demonstrating fetal cardiac activity. *J Ultrasound Med* 12(7): 383–386.

Kelly MK, Schneider EP, Petrikovsky BM & Lesser ML (2000) Effect of antenatal steroid administration on the biophysical profile. *JCU* 28: 224–226.

Lupo VR (1989) The biophysical profile. *Semin US CT and MRI* 10: 405–416.

Manning FA (1990) The use of sonography in the evaluation of high risk pregnancy. *Radiol Clin North Am* 28: 205–217.

Manning F, Morrison I, Lang I et al (1985) Fetal assessment based on fetal biophysical profile scoring. Experience in 12 620 referred high-risk pregnancies. *Am J Obstet Gynecol* 151: 343–350.

Petrikovsky BM, Oleschuk C, Lesser M et al (1997) Prediction of fetal macrosomia using sonographically measured abdominal subcutaneous tissue thickness. *JCU* 25: 378–382.

Stefos TI, Lolis DE, Sotiriadis AJ, Ziakas GV (1998) Embryonic heart rate in early pregnancy. *JCU* 26: 33–36.

Ventzileos AM, Campbell WA & Rodis JF (1994) Fetal assessment by ultrasonography. The fetal biophysical profile. In: Callen PW (ed.) *Ultrasonography in Obstetrics and Gynecology,* 3rd edn, pp 487–502, Philadelphia: WB Saunders.

Patients at Risk of Intrauterine Growth Retardation

- Previous child with growth retardation or pre-eclampsia

- Maternal illness
  Hypertension: essential or of pregnancy
  Diabetes mellitus
  Collagen vascular disease (SLE)
  Cardiac disease: particularly if causing maternal polycythemia
  Renal disease
  Sickle cell disease
  Drug addiction
  Heavy smoker
  Alcohol abuse
  Infection

- Multiple pregnancy
  Has an increased risk of IUGR, premature delivery and PH

Causes of Asymmetrical Intrauterine Growth Retardation

This is when the head circumference is less affected than the abdominal circumference.

- Idiopathic: probably due to placental failure
- Placental failure
- Maternal hypertension with proteinuria: may also be secondary to placental insufficiency
- Severe maternal illness, including cardiac disease, particularly those causing polycythemia
- Multiple gestation
- All causes of symmetric IUGR (most of the causes of symmetric IUGR may also cause asymmetric IUGR)

NB Asymmetric IUGR results from an attempt to protect vital structures at the expense of less critical organs. Of small-for-gestational-age babies, 80% have no known risk factors. Only 50% of cases are detected by clinical examination. IUGR is a significant cause of morbidity and mortality in the first year of life.

Problems Associated with Asymmetrical Growth Retardation

- **Fetal death/stillbirth**
- Intrauterine/perinatal asphyxia and hypoxia causing cerebral palsy, mental handicap, etc.
- Premature delivery
- Problems in the neonatal period
  Hypoglycemia
  Thrombocytopenia
  Pulmonary hemorrhage
  Necrotizing enterocolitis
  Hypocalcemia
  Hypothermia
  Polycythemia

NB The 'starved' fetus has low glycogen and other energy stores and is thus less able to withstand the stress of delivery and the neonatal period.

Causes of Symmetrical Intrauterine Growth Retardation

- Chromosomal anomalies
- **TORCH infections**
- Toxoplasmosis
  Rubella
  Cytomegalovirus and other viral infections
  Syphilis
- **Major maternal illness** (including collagen vascular disease)
- **Early onset placental insufficiency**
- Maternal smoking
- Structural fetal abnormality
- Idiopathic
- Maternal drug abuse
- Maternal weight below the 10th percentile for height or below 45 kg
- Sickle cell disease
- Recurrent antepartum hemorrhage
- Fetal alcohol syndrome
- Starvation
- Exposure to excessive ionizing radiation

NB Symmetrical growth retardation is said to be present when the fetus is small-for-dates (at or below the 5th percentile) but normally proportioned. In suspected IUGR an abnormal umbilical artery pulsatility index (PI) is a better predictor of adverse perinatal outcome as compared to middle cerebral artery PI. However a normal middle cerebral artery PI may identify fetuses without a major adverse perinatal outcome especially before 32 weeks gestation.

Further Reading

Fong KW, Ohlsson A, Hannah ME et al (1999) Prediction of perinatal outcome in fetuses suspected to have intra-uterine growth retardation: Doppler US study of fetal cerebral, renal and umbilical arteries. *Radiology* 213: 681–689.

Problems of Children with Symmetrical Growth Retardation

- Increased risk of death in the first year after delivery
- Reduced intellect
- Learning difficulties
- Short stature
- Chromosomal or other underlying fetal abnormality
- Complications of intrauterine infections

Conditions Associated with Elevated Maternal Serum α-Fetoprotein

Factors influencing MOM calculations

The multiples of median value of MSAFP that define normal and abnormal usually lies between 2 MOM and 3 MOM. Values are adjusted for gestational age, obesity (lower MSAFP), black women (MSAFP levels 10–15% higher than non-blacks) and maternal insulin-dependent diabetes (lower MSAFP).

Misdated pregnancy

MSAFP values vary with gestational age. They rise, reaching a peak at approximately 30 weeks gestation. The amniotic fluid AFP peaks around 12 weeks gestation. Approximately 20% of raised MSAFP levels are related to inaccurate dating, usually relating to LMP.

Multiple gestation

Twin pregnancy gives rise to approximately twice the concentration of MSAFP as singleton pregnancy. Twin pregnancy does not usually affect amniotic AFP. One should remember that the twin may be concordant or discordant for the presence of congenital anomaly associated with an elevated AFP.

Dying/recently dead fetus

Both MSAFP and amniotic fluid AFP are elevated. The cause of the elevation is unclear but may be related to loss of skin and membrane integrity.

Normal pregnancy

In many cases it is impossible to find a cause for a raised MSAFP; however, it should be noted that there is an increased prevalence of pre-natal mortality and morbidity among mothers with elevated MSAFP reflecting placental insufficiency.

Bleeding in normal pregnancy

IUGR

Placental insufficiency in the third trimester is often associated with a raised MSAFP screening test.

Open fetal defects

These include: (1) anencephaly; (2) exancephaly; (3) encephalocele; (4) spina bifida; (5) omphalocele; (6) gastroschisis; (7) bladder extrophy; (8) cloacal extrophy; (9) ectopia cordis; and (10) limb-body wall complex. These lesions may either be covered by a membrane or fully exposed to AF. There is an increased diffusion of AFP from the open surface into AFP. This high level of AFP is reflected in MSAFP. Sacrococcygeal teratoma, skin defects, epignathus, pilonidal sinus and ABS can be added to the list of open defects. MSAFP levels are usually normal in the presence of a cystic hygroma. Occasionally the hygroma may rupture, which leads to AFP-rich lymphatic fluid in the AF.

Fetomaternal

The increase in MSAFP depends upon the size of the fetomaternal hemorrhage. After amniocentesis there may be transient elevation of MSAFP, probably related to fetomaternal hemorrhage.

Renal anomalies

These include: (1) renal agenesis; (2) congenital nephrosis; (3) polycystic kidney; (4) urinary tract obstruction. Congenital nephrosis is rare except in Finland. Antenatal US diagnosis of congenital nephrosis is difficult due to lack of specific features. In mothers with very elevated MSAFP in whom an open fetal defect has been excluded on ultrasound, congenital nephrosis should be considered and an amniocentesis performed.

Placenta and AF	These include: (1) chorioangioma; (2) placental abnormalities hematoma; (3) umbilical cord hematoma or hemangioma; (4) OH.
Fetal liver abnormalities	These include: (1) liver necrosis; (2) liver tumour.
Maternal liver disease	Hepatomas and hepatitis.

Further Reading

Larson JM, Pretorius DH, Budovick NE & Scioscia AL (1993) Value of maternal serum α-fetoprotein levels of 5.0 MOM or greater and prenatal sonography in predicting fetal outcome. *Radiology* 189(1): 77–81.

Miller CE (1993) Elevated maternal serum AFP and normal ultrasound: what next? *Semin US CT MRI* 14: 31–29.

Nyberg DA, Mahoney BS, Pretorius DH et al (1991) *Diagnostic Ultrasound of Fetal Anomalies: Text and Atlas*, p. 71. Chicago: Year Book Medical.

Seeds JW & WJ (1990) Ultrasound and maternal serum feto-protein screening: a complementary relationship. *Ultrasound Q 9*: 145–166.

Ultrasound Diagnosis of Zygosity

Dizygotic Twins (2 Zygotes)

Dichorionic diamniotic	Thick separating membrane
	Separate placenta
	May be different sex
	'Delta sign' – triangular extension of placental tissue between layers of dividing membranes.

Monozygotic Twins (1 Zygote)

Dichorionic monoamniotic (1%)	Thin separating membrane
	Single placenta
	Single sex

NB Non-visualization of dividing membrane does not guarantee that the gestations are monoamniotic. Membranes may be invisible, e.g., late pregnancy or severe OH in one of the sacs ('stuck twin'). Diagnosis of zygosity is best performed in the first trimester.

Mortality Rates in Twin Pregnancy

DC + DA   9%
MC + DA   26%
MC + MA   50%

Chorionicity is most accurately assessed by US before 10 weeks gestation, although assessment up to 14 weeks is said to be acceptable. Monozygotic twins are at greater risk than dizygotic twins because

- Sixty-six percent are monochorionic and have a risk of vascular anastamosis.
- They have a higher incidence of structural anomalies.

Placentation

Each zygote from separate ova implants separately with their own chorion and amniotic cavity. Thus dizygotic twins always have a dichorionic diamniotic placentation with each twin having its own placenta. In a monozygotic twin the type of placentation depends upon the time of division of the zygote:

< 4 days after conception: Dichorionic diamniotic
4-7 days after conception: Monochorionic diamniotic
> 8 days after conception: Monochorionic monoamniotic.

Further Reading

Bronstein R, Goyent G & Bottoms S (1989) Classification of twins and neonatal morbidity. *Obstet Gynecol* 74: 98-101.

Guaschino S, Spinillo A, Stola E et al (1987) Growth retardation size at birth and perinatal mortality in twin pregnancy. *Int J Gynaecol Obstet* 25: 399-403.

Kurtz AB, Wapner RJ, Mata J et al (1992) Twin pregnancies: accuracy of first trimester abdominal US in predicting chorionicity and amnionicity. *Radiology* 155: 205-209.

Rodis JF, Vintzeleas AM, Campbell WA et al (1987) Antenatal diagnosis and management of mono-amniotic twins. *Am J Obstet Gynecol* 157: 1255-1263.

Ultrasound Determination of Chorionicity

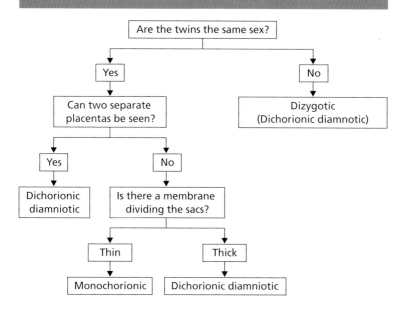

In 66% of dichorionic twins the placentas abut each other or are fused. Best assessed in the first trimester; progressively less accurate with advancing pregnancy.

Further Reading

Brass VA, Benacerraf BR & Trigoletto FD Jr (1985) Ultrasonographic determination of chorion type in twin gestation. *Obstet Gynecol* 66: 779–783.

Finberg HJ (1992) The 'twin peak' sign. Reliable evidence of dichorionic twinning. *J Ultrasound Med* 11: 571–577.

Hertzberg BS, Kurtz AB, Choi HY et al (1987) Significance of membrane thickness in the sonographic evaluation of twin gestations. *AJR* 148: 151–153.

Townsend RW, Simpson GF & Filly RA (1989) Membrane thickness in ultrasound prediction of chorionicity of twin gestations. *J Ultrasound Med* 7: 327–332.

Twin-Twin Transfusion Syndrome Versus Intrauterine Growth Retardation of One Twin

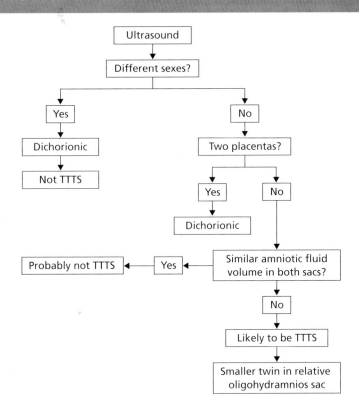

Further Reading

Brown DL, Benson CB, Driscoll SG et al (1989) Twin-twin transfusion syndrome. Sonographic findings. *Radiology* 170: 61–63.

Hecher K, Ville Y & Nicolaides KH (1995) Fetal arterial Doppler studies in twin-twin transfusion syndrome. *J Ultrasound Med* 14: 101–108.

Pretorious DH, Manchester D, Balken S et al (1988) Doppler ultrasound of the twin transfusion syndrome. *J Ultrasound Med* 14: 117–124.

Sharma S, Gray S, Guzman ER et al (1995) Detection of twin-twin transfusion by first trimester ultrasonography. *J Ultrasound Med* 14: 635–637.

Causes of Increased Risks of Twin Pregnancy

- The intrauterine fetal death rate is seven times higher than in singleton pregnancy – risk lowest for DC, DA twins and highest for MC MA twins 9%, 25% & 50% respectively. There are an increasing number of potential complications with greater sharing of membranes. While only small proportions of all pregnancies are multiple, they account for 12% of neonatal deaths.

- Twins identified in the first trimester: live born twins in 80%, singleton at delivery 9%, miscarriage 11%.

- The first twin prognosis depends on placentation type: MC gestation worse prognosis than DC ones, US may show a subchorionic haematoma or fibroids. Prognosis also depends on gestation age, with a twin pregnancy at 6 weeks gestation it is more likely to result in the loss of the entire pregnancy or deliver a singleton than at 12 weeks gestation.

- MC twins at risk of vascular complications through shared placenta, including twin-twin transfusion syndrome and acardiac twinning.

- MC MA twins have an increased risk of cord accidents such as cord entanglement.

- Monozygotic twins have an increased risk of fetal anomalies not unique to twins, which appear 3–7 times more frequently than in dizygotic twins or singletons. The anomalies that may occur in mono-zygotic twins include with increasing frequency: hydrocephalus, anencephaly, holoprosencephaly, SCT & others. The anomalies are frequently discordant, in spite of identical twins.

- Death of one twin in the first trimester may occur with no evidence on follow-up scans that there was ever evidence of a twin.

- Death of one twin in the second trimester may result in a macerated and compressed fetus against the uterine wall and may be visible on US as a paper thin structure – 'fetus papyraceus.'

- Death of one twin in the late second or third trimester: degree of maceration of the dead fetus depends upon the amount of time lapsed between death and delivery.

- High incidence of premature labor complicated by immature lungs and cerebral hemorrhage.

- Low birthweight – IUGR and placental anomalies unique to multiple gestation. All twins are at a risk of IUGR. IUGR occurs in 25–30% of twins.

- Increased incidence of polyhydramnios and oligohydramnios (7% of twins).

- Increased incidence of congenital anomalies (7%).

- Fetal interlocking malpresentation.
- Increased incidence of umbilical cord insertion anomalies.
- Increased maternal complications, particularly
  Antepartum hemorrhage
  Pregnancy-induced hypertension
  Pre-eclampsia
  Iron deficiency anemia
  Hyperemesis
  Pyelonephritis
  Cholestatis.

Sonographic surveillance of these high-risk pregnancies should be routine because early diagnosis of complications leads to better management and a reduction in fetal mortality.

Further Reading

Benson CB & Doubilet PM (1998) Multiple gestation *Ultrasound Q* 14: 234–246.
Harrison SD, Dale R, Patten CRM & Mack A (1993) Twin growth problems: causes and sonographic analysis. *Semin US CT MRI* 14: 56–67.

Fetal Anomalies Associated with Twin Pregnancy

An increased incidence of congenital malformation is seen in up to 7% of twin gestations (compared to 3% in singletons). The anomalies usually affect only one twin, although the incidence of chromosomal abnormalities in monozygotic twinning with different phenotypes should always be considered.

- CNS abnormalities, including neural tube defect, hydrocephalus, holoprosencephaly
- Congenital heart disease
- Chromosomal abnormality
- Cloacal extrophy
- Sacrococcygeal teratoma
- Sirenomelia

Further Reading

Ghai V & Vidyasagar D (1988) Morbidity and mortality factors in twins: an epidemiological approach. *Clin Perinatol* 15: 123.

Hendricks CH (1966) Twinning in relation to birthweight, mortality and congenital anomalies. *Obstet Gynecol* 27: 47–53.

Types of Conjoined Twins

Incomplete separation of fetuses, such fetuses are monochorionic and monoamniotic with an incidence of 1 in 52 000 births.

- Thoracopagus – joined at thorax 70%
- Omphalopagus – anterior abdominal wall
- Craniopagus – skull
- Pyopagus – buttocks and sacrum
- Ischiopagus – ischium
- Diprosopus – two faces

Ultrasound diagnosis

- Separate fetuses with a constant point of connection.
- Absent dividing membranes.
- Umbilical arteries may have differing Doppler waveform.
- Associated anomalies, particularly in diprosopus.

Further Reading

Barth R, Filly R, Goldberg J et al (1990) Conjoined twins: prenatal diagnoses and assessment of associated malformations. *Radiology* 177: 201.

Cohen HL, Shapiro ML, Hallen JO & Schwartz D (1992). The multi-vessel umbilical cord: an antenatal indicator of possible conjoined twinning. *JCU* 20: 278–282.

Skupski DW, Streltzoff J, Hutson M et al (1995) Early diagnosis of conjoined twins in triplet pregnancy after in utero fertilization and assisted hatching. *J Ultrasound Med 14*: 611–615.

Abnormalities Unique to Multiple Gestations

Intrauterine death of one twin	Usually occurs in the first trimester, although can occur at a later stage. The loss rate of one twin is about 20%. Diagnosis is frequently sonographic – the 'vanishing twin.' If the fetus is lost in the second trimester it may become mummified – fetus papyraceus. Loss in later pregnancy results in significant fetal loss or handicap in the surviving twin if monozygotic.
Twin-twin transfusion syndrome	This occurs in MC twins due to arteriovenous anastamosis in the shared placenta. The donor twin is small and anemic. The recipient is polycythemic and large, being at risk of high output cardiac failure. The mortality rate is 40–90% with both twins at risk. There is improved perinatal outcome with serial amnio-centeses with survival rates quoted between 37–83%, although there is a 1.5–8% complica-tion rate from large volume amniocenteses. US findings include: (1) discordance in fetal weight 25%; (2) discordance in amniotic fluid volume; PH in one sac and OH in the second sac – 'stuck twin;' (3) fetal hydrops in 10–25% of recipient twin; (4) disparity in the relative size and number of cord vessels; (5) single placenta with areas of disparity in the echogenicity of the cotyledons supplying the two cords; (6) same sex fetuses; (7) inability to visualize the donor's bladder, the recipient's bladder is enlarged.

Acardiac twinning

Occurs in 1% of MC twins; one fetus develops without a functioning heart and other severe body deformities are associated. The most common variety is absent head and heart – acardius acephalus. US reveals a twin pregnancy: one fetus has an absent or rudimentary heart; other anomalies may be present. Diffuse skin thickening is usually seen. In the acardiac twin the umbilical cord often has one artery and one vein. Reversed direction of flow can be shown by Doppler US. US helps in management by looking for evidence of heart failure in the normal twin. Early delivery can be arranged if there is fetal compromise, if lung maturity is evident.

Abnormalities in structure and blood flow

Twin embolization

Death of an MC twin may be associated with thrombotic or embolic episodes in the live twin through vascular connections in a mono-chorionic placenta. The thromboembolic material originates from the dead fetus and passes into the live fetus via intra-placental vascular connections. This results in neurologic deficit (ventriculomegaly, porencephaly and progressive thinning of the cerebral cortex) and vascular damage to the kidneys (infarcted lesions) and small bowel (calcification). Sonographic follow-up suggests that it is possible to recognize this sequential embolic phenomenon, which appears to be multiple recurrent events rather than a single event with multiple foci.

Further Reading

Bronstein R, Goyent G & Bottoms S (1998) Classification of twins and neonatal mortality. *Obstet Gynecol* 74: 98–101.

Coleman BG, Brumbach K, Arger PH et al (1987) Twin gestation monitoring of complications and anomalies with US. *Radiology* 165: 449–453.

Cook TL & O'Shaughnessy R (1997) Iatrogenic creation of a monoamniotic twin gestation in severe twin-twin transfusion syndrome. *J Ultra Med* 16: 853–855.

Elchalal U, Tanos V, Bar-Oz B & Nadjari M (1997) Early second trimester twin embolization syndrome. *J Ultra Med* 16: 509–512.

Filly RA, Goldstein RB & Collen PW (1990) Monochorionic twinning sonographic assessment. *AJR* 154: 459.

Ghai V & Vidyasgar D (1988) Morbidity and mortality factors in twins: an epidemiologic approach. *Clin Perinatol* 15: 123–127.

Patten RM, Mack LA, Nyberg DA et al (1989) Twin embolization syndrome: prenatal sonographic detection and significance. *Radiology* 173: 685.

Wenstrom K & Gall SA (1988) Incidence, morbidity and mortality, and diagnosis of twin gestation. *Clin Perinatol* 15: 1–4.

Assessment of Amniotic Fluid Volume

Amniotic Fluid Index (AFI)

The uterus is divided into four quadrants. Lines of demarcation: longitudinal: linea nigra; transverse; umbilicus. The deepest vertical pocket of AF is measured in the four quadrants. The sum of the depths of AF in the four quadrants = AFI. Normograms are available.

Polyhydramnios

Qualitative measurement – mild, moderate or severe.
Quantitative measurement – single vertical pocket of AF >8 cm.
AFI 24 cm = clinically significant PH.

Oligohydramnios

Qualitative measurement – visual lack of AF, poor fluid/fetal interface and crowding of fetal parts.
Quantitative measurement – largest pocket of AF <2 cm.
AF volume <300 ml at term.
<3rd centile for gestation.

Further Reading

Carlson DE, Platt LD, Medearis AL et al (1990) Quantifiable polyhydramnios: diagnosis and management. *Obstet Gynecol* 75: 989-992.

Hashimoto BE, Kramer DJ & Brennan L (1993) Amniotic fluid volume: fluid dynamics and measurement technique. *Semin US CT MRI* 14: 40-55.

Magann EF, Whitworth NS, Klausen JH et al (1995) Accuracy of ultrasonography in evaluating amniotic fluid volume at less than 24 weeks gestation. *J Ultrasound Med* 14: 895-897.

Meyer WJ, Font GE, Gauthier DW et al (1995) Effect of amniotic fluid volume on ultrasonic fetal weight estimation. *J Ultrasound Med* 14: 193-197.

Phelan JP, Smith CV, Broussard P et al (1987) Amniotic fluid volume assessment with four-quadrant technique at 36-42 weeks gestation. *J Reprod Med* 32: 540-542.

Rutherford SE, Smith CV, Phelan JP et al (1987) Four-quadrant assessment of amniotic fluid volume. Interobserver and intraobserver variations. *J Reprod Med* 32: 587-589.

Causes of Oligohydramnios

IUGR

- Fetal causes
  Infection
  Chromosomal abnormalities
  Fetal syndromes

- Maternal causes (systemic)
  Pre-eclampsia
  Hypertension
  Chronic cardiac, renal, GIT disease
  Connective tissue disorders, e.g. SLE
  Hemoglobinopathy

- Maternal causes (drugs)
  Indomethacin: has been used not only to inhibit preterm labor but also to reduce AF volume in multiple gestations with PH. OH is an acknowledged side effect of indomethacin.

- Maternal causes (placental)
  Placental insufficiency
  Failure of development
  Multiple infarcts
  Partial abruption

- Post-term pregnancy

- **Preterm rupture of membranes**

- Fetal demise

Fetal Abnormalities

- Obstructive uropathy (all causes extrinsic/intrinsic, e.g. prune belly syndrome, PUJ obstruction, caudal regression, absent urethra, etc.)
- Renal agenesis
- Multicystic kidney; bilateral
- Polycystic disease; infantile
- Cardiovascular
- Impending fetal death.

Causes of Polyhydramnios

Idiopathic

In 60–70% of pregnancies complicated by PH no fetal or maternal abnormality is present.

Maternal abnormality

Diabetes mellitus
Obesity
Rhesus incompatibility
Anemia
Congestive cardiac failure
Syphilis

Fetal abnormalities

(a) Large fetus

Large fetuses even when not associated with maternal diabetes mellitus can cause mild/moderate PH. This association suggests that idiopathic PH represents an over-hydrated state of a larger than expected fetus.

(b) Twin

This is commonly related to twin-twin pregnancy transfusion in monochorionic twins. An acute PH has been described, characterized by rapid accumulation of AF resulting in termination or fetal demise. In 'stuck twin' one sac may have PH while the other has OH. PH may be associated with conjoined twins.

(c) CNS abnormalities.

Usually occur in the third trimester

Anencephaly

Single most common fetal anomaly causing PH.

Hydrocephalus

84% of fetuses with hydrocephalus have other associated abnormalities.

Holoprosencephaly

Absence of falx and fusion of the thalami differentiates from other forms of fetal hydrocephalus.

Encephalocele

Hydranencephaly	Absence of forebrain and replacement by CSF as a result of an in-utero vascular accident.
Neural tube defect	Meningocele.
Dandy-Walker malformation	Usually with associated abnormalities.
Agenesis of corpus callosum	Usually with associated abnormalities.
Lissencephaly	

(c) CVS abnormalities

Fetofetal transfusion syndrome	Most common syndrome associated with PH in twin pregnancy.
Fetal hydrops	Both immune and non-immune.
Cardiac arrhythmias	Usually resulting in cardiac failure.
Myocardial disorders	
Umbilical cord knots	
Ventricular septal defects	
Coarctation of aorta	
Interruption of fetal aorta	
Trancus arteriosus	
Ectopia cordis	
Placental chorioangioma	
High output lesions, e.g. teratoma	

(d) Thoracic abnormalities **Cystic-adenomatoid malformation**

Primary pulmonary hypoplasia

Diaphragmatic hernia

Congenital chylothorax

Mediastinal/lung mass, e.g. teratoma

Tracheal atresia

Thymic hypoplasia

Pulmonary sequestration

(e) GIT abnormalities — Any condition that impairs swallowing may be associated with PH, including structural abnormalities such as cleft lip and palate, bowel atresia and neuromuscular disorders such as myotonic dystrophy.

Cleft lip and palate

Esophageal, duodenal and jejunal atresias — Atresia of distal bowel may present as multiple dilated loops of bowel. It is important to differentiate these from hydronephrotic kidneys.

VACTERAL

Congenital pancreatic cysts — May cause compression/obstruction of bowel.

Omphalocele — PH is presumably secondary to small bowel obstruction.

Gastroschisis — It is important to differentiate this entity from omphalocele because of a better prognosis.

Annular pancreas — May cause compression/obstruction of duodenum.

Meconium peritonitis

Bowel perforation

Craniolingual teratoma

Hepatic tumors

Megacystis–microcolon–intestinal hypoperistalsis syndrome

Congenital chloride diarrhea	Appearances similar to intestinal obstruction are seen.

(f) Musculoskeletal abnormalities

Achondroplasia – homozygous

Arthrogryposis

Osteogenesis imperfecta

Hypophosphatasia

Short rib-polydactyly

Asphyxiating thoracic dystrophy

Platyspondyly

Camptomelic dwarfism

Thanatophoric dwarfism

(g) Urinary tract anomalies	Usually result in oligohydramnios and urinary ascites from ruptured bladder or kidneys in bladder outflow obstruction.

Vesicoureteric reflux

Ureteropelvic junction obstruction

Congenital mesoblastic nephroma

(h) Infections*

    Coxsackie

    Toxoplasmosis

    Cytomegalovirus

    Parvovirus

    Syphilis

    *Infections may be associated with non-immune FH.

(i) Metabolic disorders*

    Inborn errors of metabolism

    Gaucher's disease

    Gangliosidosis

    Mucopolysaccharidosis

    Gangliosidosis (GM1)

    *These conditions are likely to be associated with non-immune FH.

(j) Chromosomal anomalies

Trisomy 16–18	The most common trisomy associated with PH is trisomy 18.
Trisomy 13–15	
Trisomy 21	
45X	Associated with cystic hygroma (nuchal) ascites and FH.
4p–	Associated with microcephaly, several skeletal dysplasias, CNS anomalies, diaphragmatic hernia and intestinal malrotation.

(k) Hematological abnormalities

Anemia or polysplenia	This may be related to bleeding or haemolysis.

(l) Neck masses

They may cause extrinsic compression of the esophagus and impairment of swallowing.

Cystic hygroma	Often associated with chromosomal abnormalities.
Cervical teratoma	PH may be related to obstruction and/or a high output lesion giving rise to FH. It appears as a solid/cystic mass with punctate calcification.
Congenital goiter	Solid symmetrical anterior neck mass.

(m) Miscellaneous conditions

Sacrococcygeal teratoma	May have a similar appearance to myelo-meningocele; differentiation can be made by demonstrating an anterior pelvic mass and an intact spine.
Ovarian cyst	This may cause intestinal obstruction, which may be incomplete or intermittent.
Lethal multiple pterygium syndrome	Associated with neck webs, skeletal dysplasia, genital and palatal anomalies.
ABS	PH may be related to GIT obstruction or CNS abnormalities.
Roberts' syndrome	May be associated with cleft lip/palate, skeletal dysplasias and genital abnormalities.
Noonan's syndrome	Associated with multiple system abnormalities but contributory factors towards PH include GIT, renal anomalies, chylothorax, nuchal cystic hygroma and skeletal dysplasias.

Beckwith–Wiedemann syndrome	Associated with macroglossia, omphalocele, organomegaly and microcephaly.
IUGR	IUGR usually cause OH, rarely PH may occur in association with IUGR, which is said to represent an ominous combination. The majority of fetuses have major anomalies or chromosomal defects, even if sonographic abnormalities are not detectable.

Further Reading

Barkin SZ, Pretorious DH, Beckett MD et al (1987) Severe polyhydramnios: incidence of anomalies. *AJR* 148: 155–159.

Carlson DE, Platt LD, Medearis AL et al (1990) Quantifiable polyhydramnios: diagnoses and management. *Obstet Gynecol* 75: 989–992.

Damato N, Filly RA, Goldstein RB et al (1993) Frequency of fetal anomalies in sonographically detected polyhydramnios. *J Ultrasound Med* 12: 11–15.

Hashimoto BE, Kramer DJ & Brennan L (1993) Amniotic fluid volume: fluid dynamics and measurement technique. *Semin US CT MRI* 14(1): 40–55.

Hill LM, Lazebnik N & Many A (1996) Effects of indomethacin on individual amniotic fluid indices in multiple gestation. *J Ultra Med* 15: 395–399.

Landy HJ, Isada NB & Larsen JW (1987) Genetic implications of idiopathic hydramnios. *Am J Obstet Gynecol* 157: 114–117.

Sickler GK, Nyberg DA, Sohaey R & Luthy DA (1997) Polyhydramnios and fetal intra-uterine growth restriction: ominous combination. *J Ultra Med* 16: 609–614.

Sivit CJ, Hill MC, Larsen JW et al (1987) Second-trimester polyhydramnios: evaluation with US. *Radiology* 165: 467–469.

Sivit CJ, Hill MC & Larsen JW (1989) Ultrasound evaluation of amniotic fluid disorders. *Ultrasound Q* 7: 39–72.

Sohaey R (1998) Amniotic fluid and umbilical cord: The fetal milieu and lifeline. *Semin Ultrasound CT & MRI* 19: 355–369.

Twinning P (1992) Value of transvaginal scanning in the assessment of second trimester oligohydramnios. *Br J Radiol* 65 (773): 455–457.

High Level Echoes in Amniotic Fluid

Described as a 'cloud of echogenic floating flakes,' homogeneously echogenic, very echogenic, or sludge-like AF.

Vernix caseosa

Meconium staining   Can give a 'snowstorm' appearance.

Intra-amniotic
hemorrhage

Denudation skin   Skin particles floating in amniotic fluid –
disorders   'snowflake' sign.

Normal variant

Further Reading

Meizner I & Carmi RL (1990) The 'snowflake sign'. A sonographic marker for prenatal detection of fetal skin denudation. *J Ultrasound Med* 9: 607.

Petrikovsky B, Schneider EP & Gross B (1998) Clinic significance of echogenic amniotic fluid. *JCU* 26: 191–193.

Assessment of Fetal Hydrops

A variety of conditions, varying from those that are incompatible with life to those that are amenable to treatment, are associated with hydrops fetalis. Sonography has an important role in the evaluation of this disorder. The following maternal and fetal features are assessed for their presence and extent.

- Fetal ascites, pleural effusion or pericardial effusion
- Skin thickness (fetal anasarca)
- Maternal hydramnios or oligohydramnios
- Abnormally thick placenta >6 cm
- Fetal heart rate and rhythm
- Search for fetal anatomical abnormality
- Consider karyotyping procedure

Causes of Fetal Hydrops

This is defined as skin oedema and fluid in one other potential space, e.g. pericardial, pleural or peritoneal.

Immune	Secondary hemolysis of fetal cells by maternal antibodies, e.g. Rhesus disease, Kell antibodies.
Cardiovascular	Arrhythmias, both tachyarrhythmias and heart block. Anatomic defects – hypoplastic left heart, Ebstein anomaly, pulmonary, aortic atresia, etc. Cardiomyopathy Endocardial fibroelastosis Myocarditis (coxsackievirus, CMV) Tumor – rhabdomyoma Congenital left ventricular aneurysm Myocardial infarction Idiopathic arterial calcification.
Pulmonary	Diaphragmatic hernia Cystic adenomatoid malformation Chylothorax Pulmonary sequestration Tracheal atresia Bronchogenic cysts Intrapulmonary tumors.
Chromosomal	Trisomy 21 Turner's syndrome Triploidy.

Hematologic	α-Thalassemia: autosomal recessive with a recurrence rate for subsequent pregnancies. It is a major cause of non-immune hydrops fetalis in the Far-East. The condition is uniformly fatal associated with a significant risk of maternal morbidity. α-Thalassemia gene is found in 20–30% of the population of the Southeast Asia. The pathophysiology includes anemia, hypo-proteinemia, portal hypertension and high output cardiac failure. Early prenatal diagnosis is vital because of the uniformly fatal fetal outcome. Sonographic features: edematous placenta and cord, hepatosplenomegaly, ascites, cardiomegaly, pericardial effusion, OH, sub-cutaneous edema, decreased fetal movement, enlarged umbilical veins and pleural effusions. Most of these signs appear late in the second or third trimester. Early US features include fetal ascites, increased placental size, hepato-splenomegaly and dilated umbilical veins. The latter is usually rather subjective and may not be obvious until 25–28 weeks gestation. If suspected DNA analysis of fetal tissue by chorionic villous sampling, amniocenteses or cordiocentesis is diagnostic
	Red cell enzyme disorders – glucose isomerase, pyruvate and 6GDP deficiency Congenital leukemia Fanconi anemia Congenital dyserthropoietic anemia Fetal and feto-maternal hemorrhage Kasabach–Merrit syndrome.

Infections	CMV
	Toxoplasmosis
	Parvovirus B19
	Adenovirus
	Rubella
	Coxsackievirus
	Herpes simplex
	Respiratory syncytial virus
	Listeria monocytogenes
	Chlamydia trachomatis
	Syphilis
	Influenza B.
Neoplastic	Neuroblastoma
	Teratoma
	Congenital leukemia.
Genitourinary	Severe obstructive uropathy
	Renal vein thrombosis.
Liver	Hepatic fibrosis
	Hepatic vascular abnormality
	Hemangioendothelioma
	Hemochromatosis: uncommon cause of HF however if ascites is seen in the fetus it may be worthwhile to evaluate the hepatic surface for nodularity and thus cirrhosis as a part of evaluation of the fetus for a cause of the disease. Findings in fetal cirrhosis: OH, cardiomegaly, diffuse
	Thickening of the skin, ascites, FH and nodularity of hepatic surface.
GIT	Meconium peritonitis/perforation
	Fetal volvulus.
Metabolic	Gaucher's disease
	Gangliosidosis
	Hurler's syndrome
	Mucolipidosis.
Cranial	Vein of Galen aneurysm.

Skeletal	Achondroplasia
	Achondrogenesis
	Osteogenesis imperfecta
	Thanatophoric dysplasia
	Short rib-polydactyly syndrome
	Asphyxiating thoracic dysplasia
	Conradi's syndrome.
Muscular	Pena–Shokeir syndrome
	Pterygium syndrome
	Arthrogryposis multiplex.
Syndromes (genetic)	Noonan's
	Neu-Laxova
	Opitz-Frias
	Cornelia de Lange
	Mohr
	Elejade
	Angio-osteohypertrophy.
Maternal	Severe anemia
	Hypoproteinemia.

Further Reading

Cyr DR, Guntheroth WG, Nyberg DA et al (1988) Prenatal diagnosis of an intra-pericardial teratoma: a cause for non-immune hydrops. *J Ultrasound Med* 7: 87.

Fleischer AC, Killam AP, Boehm FH et al (1981) Hydrops fetalis: sonographic evaluation and clinical implications. *Radiology* 141: 163–168.

Fleming P & McLeary RD (1987) Non-immunologic fetal hydrops with theca lutein cysts. *Radiology* 141: 169–170.

Graves GR & Basket TF (1984) Non-immune hydrops fetalis: antenatal diagnosis and management. *Am J Obstet Gynecol* 150: 805.

McGahan JP & Schneider J (1986) Fetal neck hemangioendothelioma with secondary hydrops fetalis. Sonographic diagnosis. *JCU* 14: 393.

Thomas CS, Leopold GR, Hilton S et al (1986) Fetal hydrops associated with extralobar pulmonary sequestration. *J Ultrasound Med* 6: 688.

Tongsong T, Wanapirak C, Srisomboon J et al (1996) Antenatal sonographic features of 100 alpha-thalassemia hydrops fetalis fetuses. *JCU* 24: 73–77.

Consequences of Amniotic Band Syndrome

Sonography may show an aberrant band or sheet of tissue attached to the fetus with secondary deformity. Even when a band is not visualized the non-embryological distribution of the abnormalities is highly suggestive of the diagnosis of ABS. The manifestations of ABS are protean and any part of the fetal body may be affected/amputated.

Head	Clefts
	Encephalocele
	Calvarial defects
	Anencephaly
	Hydrocephalus.
Face	'Slash' defects
	Atypical facial, lip and palatal clefts.
Thorax	Slash defects with secondary deformity, e.g. exteriorization of heart
	Chest deformity – may cause secondary lung hypoplasia.
Spine	Kyphosis
	Scoliosis
	Meningomyelocele
	Other rotational anomalies
	Amputation of lower spine.
Abdomen	'Slash' defects
	Omphalocele
	Gastropleuroschisis (exteriorization of bowel, liver and heart without a covering)
	Imperforate anus.
Genitalia	Amputation
	Malformed.
Limbs	Clubfoot
	Limb constriction with elephantiasis
	Amputation
	Distal syndactyly.

Further Reading

Baker CJ & Rudolph AJ (1971) Congenital ring constrictions and intrauterine amputation. *Am J Dis Child* 212: 393.

Budorick NE, Pretorius DH, McGahan JP et al (1995) Cephalocele detection in utero: Sonographic and clinical features. *Ultrasound Obstet Gynecol* 5(2): 77–85.

Emanuel PG, Garcia GI & Angtuaco TL (1995) Prenatal detection of anterior abdominal wall defects with US. *Radiographics* 15(3): 517–530.

Fiske CE, Filly RA & Globus MS (1988) Prenatal ultrasound diagnosis of amniotic band syndrome. *J Ultrasound Med* 7: 293–295.

Mahoney B, Filly RA, Callen PW et al (1985) The amniotic band syndrome: antenatal sonographic diagnosis and potential pitfalls. *Am J Obstet Gynecol* 152: 63–68.

Malpas T, Anderson N & Langley S (1995) Ulnar club-hand and constricting-ring syndrome. *Pediatr Radiol* 25(3): 233–234.

Ossipoff V & Hall BD (1977) Etiologic factors in the amniotic band syndrome. Study of 24 patients. *Birth Defects* 13: 117.

Randall SB, Filly RA, Callen PW et al (1988) Amniotic sheets. *Radiology* 166: 633–636.

Woods T & Romonsky N (1995) Congenital constriction band syndrome. *J Am Pediatr Med Assoc* 85(6): 310–314.

Intrauterine Membranes Unassociated with Amniotic Band Syndrome

Amnion

Visualization of the amnion in the first trimester of pregnancy is of no clinical significance and is unassociated with anomalies recorded with ABS. Visualization of the amnion is a normal finding before 14 weeks gestation and should not be seen after 16 weeks gestation.

Normal separation

Separation of the amniotic from the chorio-amniotic chorionic membrane is normal in early pregnancy until fusion of the two membranes at approximately 16 weeks.

Traumatic chorioamniotic separation

This may follow amniocentesis; the process is benign and usually has no associated abnormalities. However it has been suggested that chorioamniotic separation occurring after mid-trimester genetic amniocentesis is associated with adverse fetal outcome i.e. in utero death or preterm labor. It is therefore prudent to closely follow these patients and consider early delivery if fetal distress occurs.

Extrachorionic separation

Extrachorionic hemorrhage separates the chorioamniotic membrane from the uterine wall, allowing visualization.

Diamniotic twins

In diamniotic twins the separating membrane is a well shown sonographic finding.

Septate uterus

Septate or bicornuate uterus is a congenital abnormality. The indenting tissue is usually located at the fundus and is orientated anterior to posterior. Myometrial tissue can often be seen extending into the base of the septum. Color and pulsed Doppler US using TVS reveal vascularized septa in 71%. Patients with vascularized septa have a higher prevalence of obstetric complications than avascular septa.

Asherman's syndrome

Intrauterine synechia (complete or incomplete) may follow cesarean section, myomectomy, trauma, inflammation, curettage, manual removal of the placenta, septic abortion, endometriosis, etc. Over 70% have usually had instrumentation of the endometrial cavity. The sheets seen on ultrasound consist of two layers of amnion and chorion around the scar. Fetal entrapment does not occur. Patients usually have a low pregnancy rate, but presence of synechiae detected sonographically during pregnancy does not seem to alter pregnancy outcome for malpresentation. Sonohysterography in conjunction with TVS is a useful technique for evaluating the disease. An echogenic area in the endometrial cavity or an asymmetric thickness of the endometrium on a transverse scan of the uterus is highly suggestive of the presence of intrauterine synechiae. TVS has a prognostic value, patients with endometrium <2 mm in the luteal phase do not benefit from surgery.

Amniotic sheets/shelves

These have a broad base at the uterine wall with a free bulbous edge protruding into the amniotic cavity. They are not fixed to the fetus. The fetus can move freely around the membrane and does not become deformed. Part of the placenta may be implanted on the amniotic sheet. Pregnancy outcome is similar in patients with and those without placental implantation. Differentiation is made between amniotic sheets, which comprise of two layers of chorion and amnion and are thicker than amniotic bands. Amniotic bands are made up of a single layer of amnion. Delivery occurs slightly early in patients with amniotic sheets. Fetal growth is not affected. There is an increased rate of cesarian section.

Intra-amniotic membrane following amniocentesis	Real time sonography demonstrates active bleeding if the needle penetrates the placenta/chorionic plate vessels following amniocentesis. Bleeding is visible on real time sonography as bright flakes, which float in the amniotic fluid, settling in the most dependent area of the sac. Blood may cause strings/bands stretching from the placenta to the fetus.
Blighted twin and circumvallate placenta	These are unusual causes of sonographic reflectors within the uterus but are rarely confused with ABS. Circumvallate placenta results when the chorioamniotic membrane inserts at some inward distance away from the edge of the placenta.
Harlequin ichthyosis	An autosomal recessive disorder, which is characterized by markedly thickened skin associated with fissuring that causes a diamond-shaped pattern on the skin surface. The eyelids and lips may be everted. A membrane of skin attached to the anterior abdominal wall floating in AF has been reported in the fetus. Diagnosis is achieved by skin biopsy.

Further Reading

Bell RH, Buchmeir SE & Longnecker M (1997) Clinical significance of sonographically detected uterine synechiae in pregnant patients. *J Ultra Med* 16: 465–469.

Benacerraf BR & Frigoletto FD (1992) Sonographic observations of amniotic rupture without amniotic band syndrome. *J Ultrasound Med* 11: 109–111.

Brown DL, Felker RE & Emmerson DS (1989) Intrauterine shelves in pregnancy: sonographic observations. *AJR* 153: 821–824.

Carlan SJ, Greenbaum LD, Parker JF et al (1993) Intra-amniotic membranes following amniocentesis. *J Clin Ultrasound* 21: 402–404.

Kapesic S & Kurjak A (1998) Septate uterus: detection and prediction of obstetrical complications by different forms of ultrasonography. *J Ultrasound Med* 17: 631–636.

Korbin CD, Benson CB & Doubilet PM (1998) Placental implantation on amniotic sheet: effect on pregnancy outcome. *Radiology* 206: 773–775.

Levine D, Callen PW, Pender SG et al (1998) Chorioamniotic separation after second-trimester genetic amniocentesis: Importance and frequency. *Radiology* 209: 175–181.

Meizner I (1992) Prenatal ultrasound features in a rare case of congenital ichthyosis (harlequin fetus). *JCU* 20: 132–134.

Mihalko M, Lindfors KKI, Grix AW et al (1989) Prenatal sonographic diagnosis of harlequin ichthyosis. *AJR* 153: 827–828.

Randel SB, Filly RA, Callen PW et al (1988) Amniotic sheets. *Radiology* 166: 633–636.

Salle B, Gaucherand P, Hilaire PDS & Rudigoz C (1999) Transvaginal sonohysterographic evaluation of intrauterine adhesions. *JCU* 27: 131–134.

Sauerbei EE & Pham DH (1986) Placental disruption and subchorionic hemorrhage in the first trimester of pregnancy. US appearances and clinical outcome. *Radiology* 160: 109.

Smeele B, Wamsteker K, Sarstadt T et al (1989) Ultrasonic appearances of Asherman's syndrome in the first trimester of pregnancy. *JCU* 17: 602–606.

Causes of Uterine Enlargement (Relative to Gestational Age)

Incorrect gestational age

Incorrect palpation

- Full maternal bladder

Large baby

Multiple pregnancy   When assessing gestational age by sonography the larger of the fetuses should be studied.

Polyhydramnios

Pelvic masses   e.g. fibroids, ovarian cysts.

Huge fetal masses   e.g. hydrocephalus, teratomas, etc.

Small Uterus for Gestational Age

- Incorrect gestational age
- Incorrect palpation
- Fetal death/missed abortion
- **Oligohydramnios**
- Spontaneous rupture of membranes
- Intrauterine growth retardation

Causes of Lower Abdominal Pain in Pregnancy

First and second trimester	Ectopic pregnancy
	Large corpus luteum cyst (>5 cm)
	Threatened or inevitable spontaneous abortion
	Degeneration of fibroids
	Cause unrelated to pregnancy: Appendicitis, UTI, ureteric colic, etc.
Third trimester	Abruption
	Preterm labor
	Degeneration of fibroid
	Torsion of ovary
	Cause unrelated to pregnancy (see above)
	Space-occupying mass, i.e. cyst.

Causes of Per Vaginum Bleeding in Pregnancy

First trimester   Abortion – incomplete, missed or threatened
                                Blighted ovum
                                Gestational trophoblastic disease/hydatidiform
                                mole
                                Ectopic gestation
                                Ruptured corpus luteum cyst
                                Bleeding of unknown cause
                                Cervical erosion.

Second and third   Placenta previa
trimester   Placental abruption
                                Hydatidiform mole
                                Pregnancy loss
                                Premature rupture of membranes
                                Cervical varices*.

Further reading

Huston T, Morrill HM, Mascola M & Bromley B (1998) Cervical varices: an unusual etiology for third trimester bleeding. *JCU* 26: 317–319.

* Most cervical varices have been reported in association with in utero exposure to diethylstilbestrol. TVS: tubular tubules with blood flow may be delineated with Color or pulsed Doppler imaging.

Ultrasound Appearances of Placenta

The placenta is first visible on US as a focal thickening along the periphery of the gestational sac from around 8 weeks of gestation. By the end of the first trimester it can be identified as a fine granular, disk-like structure occupying a major part of the endometrial surface. Circumferential growth occurs throughout most of pregnancy. As it matures the placenta develops a stronger echo pattern than the underlying myometrium. The chorionic plate is seen as a bright linear echo lying between the homogeneous tissue of the body of the placenta and amniotic fluid.

Gestational age (weeks)	Sonographic findings
8	Focal thickening of the gestational sac wall is first visible
12	Placenta is clearly visible in most cases. Echogenicity is initially similar to the myometrium but increases
16	Placenta and fetus are of similar size
20+	The placenta is usually 2–3 cm thick (max, normal = 4 cm; placentas more than 5 cm thick should be considered pathological)
29	Placental calcification becomes visible
33	50% of placentas now show foci of calcification

Ultrasound Grading of Placenta

The changes in placental appearances visible on US have been used to grade the placenta. The placenta is normally 3 cm thick and 15–20 cm in diameter.

Grade

0	Homogeneous placental echo pattern and a smooth chorionic plate. Grade 0 placenta is normal till 31 weeks of gestation but is not usually seen at term
I	Random echogenic foci become visible within the placental substance and subtle chorionic undulations may occur. Forty percent of placentas at term are grade I
II	More focal echogenic areas are present giving a 'comma-like' appearance. Basal densities have a stippled appearance. The chorionic plate is now becoming irregular (40% of placentas at term)
III	The chorionic plate indentations now extend deep into the placenta to the basal layers. Echogenic foci are prominent and may cause distal overshadowing. These echogenic areas may be confluent in basal area (20% of placentas at term). Reaching grade III before 31 weeks may indicate placental failure

Placental appearances have been used to assess maturity of the gestation but placental grading is an unreliable indicator of fetal lung maturity.

Further Reading

Harris RD, Cho C & Wells WA (1996) Sonography of the placenta with emphasis on pathological correlation. *Seminars in US, CT and MRI* 17(1): 66–89.

Causes of Premature Placental Aging

Maternal illness	Toxemia of pregnancy
	Hypertension
	Sickle cell anemia
	Drug abuse.
Placental abnormality	Placental failure
	Abruptio placenta
	Premature rupture of membranes.

Causes of Delayed Placental Aging

- Gestational diabetes mellitus
- Hydrops fetalis
- Multiple pregnancy.

Further Reading

Benirschke K & Kaufmann P (1990) *Pathology of the Human Placenta,* 2nd ed, pp 1–79, New York: Springer-Verlag.

Variation in Placental Morphology

Succenturiate lobe

One or more accessory lobes attached to the main placental vessels. The accessory lobe may be in previa position with its associated complications. Accessory lobes may also be retained after delivery.

Placental lakes

Large placental lakes lie in the intervillous spaces and contain moving blood.

Highly echogenic areas

Normal appearance in an aging placenta.

Placental cysts

Most cyst-like areas in the placenta are related to blood vessels. However, nonvascular placental cysts are not uncommon.

Placenta accreta

Normally there is villous invasion of the decidua. Occasionally the chorionic villi penetrate deeply into the myometrium. Placenta accreta increases the likelihood of placental retention, persistent bleeding or infections post delivery. The sonolucent area seen in the retroplacental region is lost in the accreta variety. Placenta accreta occurs in 5% of patients with placenta previa. Scarring of the uterus following cesarian section increases the prevalence of placenta previa from 0.26% in a normal uterus to 0.65% after a single cesarian section to 10% after 4 or more cesarian sections. The frequency of placenta accreta in the presence of placenta previa increases from 24% after one cesarian section to 67% after 4 cesarian sections. US reveals loss of normal retroplacental hypoechoic zone (normal > 2 mm) thinning or disruption of hyperechoic uterine serosa–bladder interface, presence of focal exophytic masses and lacunar flow within the placenta. Doppler US highlights regions of increased vascularity associated with dilated vessels that cross the placental and uterine wall and highlights transition from a normal Doppler signal in the retroplacental hypoechoic zone to that of absent Doppler signal and the myometrial zone.

Placenta increta (17%) | The villi extend through the myometrium.

Placenta percreta (5%) | The villi penetrate the uterine serosa.

Circumvallate placenta | The fetal membranes are attached to the inner aspect of the placenta instead of its edges. A depression is often seen at the point of membrane insertion, giving the appearance of a 'ditch.' This abnormality of placental shape is associated with a higher incidence of IUGR, perinatal death, placental abruption, preterm labor and fetal anomalies. The accuracy of US diagnosis of a circumvallate placenta is limited.

Battledore placenta | The umbilical cord inserts into the edge of the placenta and not the center. Rarely the cord enters in the membranes, with the vessels running through the membranes to reach the placenta.

Systemic maternal disorders | The placenta may be thickened in Rh incompatibility, gestational diabetes and mild cases of non-gestational diabetes. Systemic maternal infections (e.g. syphilis) and maternal anemia may also cause thickening. There is a higher than normal incidence of placental infarction and abruption in toxemia of pregnancy.

Placenta previa | Sonographic diagnosis depends upon the identification of placental tissue covering part or all the internal os. Placenta previa is associated with (1) increasing maternal age; (2) multiparity; (3) uterine surgery.

Classification of placental location
Grade 1 Low lying
Grade 2 Marginal previa
Grade 3 Partial previa (complete asymmetrical)
Grade 4 Complete previa (complete symmetrical)

Abnormal cord insertions   The umbilical cord normally inserts in the central portion of the placenta. The umbilical cord may be abnormally sited when it inserts at the edge of placenta – marginal cord insertion. The cord vessels may separate from each other and course between the amnion and chorion before reaching the placenta – velamentous cord insertion. Abnormal cord insertions are thought to be associated with increased perinatal mortality and morbidity such as intrapulmonary hemorrhage, still birth, fetal bradycardia IUGR, twin to twin transfusion and preterm labor. With gray scale US and Color Doppler, abnormal cord insertion can be identified. A normal cord insertion on US does not completely exclude the presence of an abnormal cord insertion on pathological examination (8%). The addition of CD improves distinction between marginal and velamentous cord insertion. Velamentous cords lack Wharton's jelly, the vessels are thinner than normal making them more difficult to identify on conventional US.

Further Reading

Di Salvo DN, Benson CB, Laing FC et al (1998) Sonographic evaluation of the placental cord insertion site. *AJR* 170: 1295–1298.

Hoffman-Tretin JC, Koenigsberg M, Robin A et al (1992) Placenta accreta: additional sonographic observations. *J Ultrasound Med* 11: 29–34.

Jauniaux E, Avni FE, Donner C et al (1989) Ultrasonic diagnosis and morphological study of placenta circumvallate. *JCU* 17: 126.

Levine D, Hulka CA, Ludmin J et al (1997) Placenta accreta: Evaluation with Color Doppler US, Power-Doppler US and MR Imaging. *Radiology* 205: 773–776.

Spirit BA & Gordon LP (1990) Sonographic evaluation of the placenta: importance of pathologic correlation. *Radiology* 176: 9.

Causes of False-Positive Ultrasound Diagnosis of Placenta Previa

Previa

This is usually due to technical artifacts.

Overfull bladder

Squashes the lower uterine segment apparently elongating the cervical canal (normally 3.5–4 cm).

Focal myometrial contraction

Uterine wall >1.5 cm thick due to Braxton-Hicks contractions. Partially empty the bladder and rescan 20–60 minutes, by which time the appearances should have changed. TVS improves the accuracy of a placental location in relating to the internal os, particularly in the posterior placenta with late gestation. As the lower uterine segment grows disproportionately to the rest of the uterus a placenta may appear to be previa in the second trimester. However scanning at 34 weeks frequently shows that this is not the case.

Placental Echo-Poor Masses

- Normal subplacental complex
- Septal cysts
- Mature placenta
- **'Maternal lakes'**
- **Intervillous thrombosis**
- **Subchorionic thrombosis**
- **Avillous spaces**
- **Placental hemorrhage**
- Subchorionic lakes
- Placental degeneration
- Hematoma (including bleed after chorionic villus sampling)
- Primary tumors: partial hydatidiform mole, chorioangioma, teratoma
- Metastases: melanoma, breast, bronchus
- Hemangioma.

Further Reading

Harris RD, Wells WA, Black WC et al (1997) Accuracy of perinatal sonography for detecting circumvallate placenta. *AJR* 168: 1603–1608.

Hertzberg BS, Bowie JD, Carrroll BA et al (1992) Diagnosis of placenta previa during the third trimester: role of transperineal sonography. *AJR* 159: 83–87.

McCarthy J, Thurmond AS, Jones MK et al (1995) Circumvallate placenta: sonographic diagnosis. *J Ultra Med* 14: 21–26.

Spirit BA & Gordon LP (1990) Sonographic evaluation of the placenta. Importance of pathologic correlation. *Radiology* 176: 9.

Retroplacental Echo-Poor Masses

- Varying degree of bladder filling can cause transient myometrial thickening
- Braxton-Hicks contractions
- **Retroplacental hemorrhage/hematoma**
- Normal placental venous drainage
- Peripheral placental infarct
- **Uterine leiomyoma**
- Myometrial hyperplasia/hypertrophy.

Causes of Chorioamniotic Separation

- Normal before 16 weeks
- Polyhydramnios
- **Amniocentesis**
- Congenital anomalies
- **Premature rupture of membranes.**

(Anechoic channels along uterine wall may be mistaken for abruptio placentae.)

Differential Diagnosis of Marginal Subchorionic Hematoma

- Placenta previa
- Succenturiate lobe
- Myoma
- Chorioangioma.

Causes of Thin Placenta

- Intrauterine growth retardation
- Toxemia of pregnancy
- Polyhydramnios
- Intrauterine infections
- Chromosomal fetal abnormality.

Causes of Placental Thickening (>4 cm)

Maternal causes

- **Maternal diabetes mellitus**
- Focal placental hemorrhage
- Placental abruption
- Normal variant
- Chronic intrauterine infection
- Maternal congestive cardiac failure
- α-thalassemia
- Moderate/severe maternal anemia of any cause.

Fetal causes

- **Rhesus sensitization**
- **Hydrops fetalis**
- Umbilical vein obstruction
- Triploidy (focal thickening or 'chronic' thickening due to secondary villous hyperplasia)
- Sacrococcygeal teratoma (associated with high output heart failure)
- **Fetal cardiac failure, particularly high output failure**
- Beckwith–Wiedemann syndrome
- Twin-twin transfusion syndrome.

Further Reading

Haddock WK, Mahoney BS, Callen PW & Filly RA (1985) Placental thickness. *J Ultrasound Med* 4: 479.

Mintz MC, Kurtz AB, Avenson R et al (1986) Abruptio placentae: apparent thickening of the placenta caused by hypoechoic retroplacental clot. *J Ultrasound Med* 5: 411.

Causes of Placental Abruption

- Maternal hypertension
- Toxemia of pregnancy
- Trauma
- Vascular disease
- Previous abruption
- Perinatal death or preterm delivery
- Short umbilical cord
- Drug abuse (e.g. cocaine)
- Smoking
- Underlying uterine or fetal malformation
- Chorioangiomas.

Ultrasound Findings in Placental Abruption

- This is a clinical diagnosis with minimal or absent ultrasound findings
- A retroplacental hematoma may appear echolucent, depending upon the age and size of hematoma
- A retroplacental hematoma may give the appearance of focal placental thickening
- Large placental hematomas may appear as solid or cystic masses
- Separation of placental margin may give the edge of the placenta a rounded appearance
- Intra-amniotic hemorrhage may give the amniotic fluid a speckled appearance
- Fluid/blood levels have been recorded within the amniotic fluid
- The fetus may swallow blood, giving rise to an echogenic mass within the stomach and echogenic bowel
- Ultrasound confirms fetal viability.

Retroplacental Hemorrhage Versus Marginal (Subchorionic) Hemorrhage

	Retroplacental	Marginal
Vaginal bleeding	Unusual	Common
Cause	Rupture of spiral arteries – 'high pressure bleed'	Tears of marginal vessels – 'low pressure bleed'
Associations	Maternal BP and vascular disease	Decidual necrosis secondary to cigarette smoking
Symptoms	'Classical' Tense, painful uterus Precipitous delivery DIC Fetal death	Often mild
Incidence	Less common	More common
Preterm labor and delivery	+	+

Further Reading

Jaffe MH, Schoen WC, Silver TM et al (1981) Sonography of abruptio placenta. *AJR* 137: 1049

McGohen JP, Phillips HE, Reid MH et al (1982) Sonographic spectrum of retroplacental hemorrhage. *Radiology* 142: 481.

Mintz MC, Kurtz AB, Aveson R et al (1986) Abruptio placentae: apparent thickening of the placenta caused by hypoechoic retroplacental clot. *J Ultrasound Med* 5: 411.

Nyberg DA, Cyr DR, Mack LA et al (1987) Sonographic spectrum of placental abruption. *AJR* 148: 161.

Walker JM & Ferguson DD (1988) The sonographic appearance of blood in the fetal stomach and its association with placental abruption. *J Ultrasound Med* 7: 155–161.

Complications of Chorioangioma

These are often incidental findings.

Maternal

Polyhydramnios
Premature labor/premature rupture of membranes
Placental abruption
May cause elevated maternal serum AFP
Toxemia of pregnancy
Postpartum hemorrhage
Retained placenta
Dystocia.

Fetal

IUGR
Intrauterine demise
Hydrops – non-immune
Prematurity
Congestive cardiac failure
Cardiomegaly
Hematologic – anemia
Microangiopathic hemolytic anemia
Thrombocytopenia
Anemia due to chronic fetal to maternal hemorrhage
May simulate a fetal tumor

Chorioangioma is the most common non-trophoblastic benign placental tumor; the incidence has been quoted as occurring in up to 1% of pregnancies. Most lesions are small and insignificant. Tumors larger than 5 cm may cause symptoms. Sonographically chorioangiomas are usually seen as well defined solid or complex solid/fluid masses protruding from the fetal surface of the placenta or lying within the placental substance. Chorioangiomas can give the appearances of a group of well circumscribed placental cysts.

Further Reading

Arodi J, Auslender R, Atad J et al (1985) Giant chorioangioma of the placenta. *Acta Obstet Gynecol Scand* 64: 90–91.

Daor AH, Rogers CW & Wong SW (1981) Chorioangioma of the placenta: report of 2 cases with ultrasound study in 1. *Obstet Gynecol* 57: 46–47.

Kedar RP, Malde HM & Jagesia DH (1994) Multiple chorioangiomas: ultrasonographic appearance, diagnosis and significance. *Can Assoc Radiol J* 45: 221–223.

Wolf BK & Wallace JHK (1987) Pitfall to avoid: chorioangioma of the placenta simulating fetal tumour. *JCU* 15: 405–408.

Zoler AH (1986) Placental chorioangioma. An unusual cause of polyhydramnios. Antenatal diagnosis. *J Can Assoc Radiol* 37: 60–611.

Vasa Previa

Vasa previa (VP) results when the placental blood vessels traverse the internal os, without the protective covering of the placenta or umbilical cord. VP carries one of the highest fetal mortalities of any complication of pregnancy, which usually remains unrecognized until the complication sets in. The exposed vessels are liable to injury and hemorrhage at the time of the rupture of the membranes. Even in the absence of hemorrhage fetal death can ensue due to hypoxia from vessel compression. VP is rare but when present, it is an absolute indication for cesarian section. Antepartum diagnosis has been achieved by transabdominal, TVS and transperineal US.

Ultrasound diagnosis

- Depends upon a high index of clinical suspicion in the appropriate clinical setting
- Sought specifically when there is a succenturiate or bilobate placenta implanted low in the uterus or a low velamentous insertion of the cord
- Curvilinear tubular structures overlying the internal os
- Color Doppler/spectral Doppler confirms the tubular structures overlying the internal os as blood vessels

Further Reading

Daley-Jones E, Hollingsworth J & Sepulveda W (1996) Vasa praevia: second trimester diagnosis using Colour flow imaging. *Br J Obstet Gynaecol* 103: 284

Hata K, Hato T, Fujiwaki R et al (1994) An accurate antenatal diagnosis of vasa previa with transvaginal Color Doppler ultrasonography. *Am J Obstet Gynecol* 171: 265.

Hertzberg BS & Kliewer MA (1998) Prenatal diagnosis by transperineal sonography with Doppler evaluation. *JCU* 28: 405–408.

Retained Placenta

Placental fragments may be retained after abortion or full-term delivery giving rise to persistent, sometimes life-threatening, post-partum hemorrhage. There is also an increased risk of infection. Retention of part or whole of the placenta particularly occur with placenta accreta and is the most common cause of morbidity of this placental anomaly.

US features

- Echogenic areas continuous with uterine wall – considered retained placenta
- Echogenic areas not continuous with the uterine wall – considered blood clot

Further Reading

de Vries JIP, van der Linden RM & van der Linden HC (2000) Predictive value of sonographic examination to visualize retained placenta directly after birth 16-28 weeks. *J Ultra Med* 19: 7-12.

Factors Affecting Fetal Umbilical Artery Waveforms

- Fetal myocardial contractility
- Fetal heart rate
- Vessel wall elasticity
- Blood viscosity
- Umbilical/placental circulation resistance
- Sample site in the umbilical cord
- Fetal breathing
- Any fetal movement

Factors Affecting Doppler Vascular Waveforms in the Fetus

Fetal respiration	Fetal respiration affects the maximum systolic and diastolic values and also affects the length of the cardiac cycle. Measurements should be taken with the fetus in a quiet non-breathing state.
Tachycardia	Heart rates over 190/min exaggerate the diastolic component of the indices by not allowing any 'run off' time.
Bradycardia	Prolonged diastole allows excessive 'run off ' time and thus diastole (max.) is artificially low.
Blood hematocrit	Decreased fetal blood hematocrit in conditions such as Rh sensitization is associated with increased fetal blood velocity.
Blood viscosity	The umbilical artery systolic:diastolic ratio increases with increasing blood velocity at high shear rates but not at low rates. Similarly a significant negative correlation exists between umbilical venous blood flow and blood viscosity.

NB   Correction methods taking heart rates into account are available.There is no significant difference in the waveforms obtained by continuous wave and pulsed wave Doppler.

Assessment of Peripheral Resistance

Qualitative   Increased resistance in peripheral vessels leads to decreased diastolic blood flow. Marked increase in peripheral resistance leads to absent or reversed diastolic blood flow.

Quantitative (angle independent methods)

Pourcelot (resistive/resistance) index

$$= \frac{\text{systolic (max.)} - \text{diastolic (min.)}}{\text{Systolic (max.)}}$$

Pulsatility index

$$= \frac{\text{systolic (max.)} - \text{diastolic (min.)}}{\text{(mean)}}$$

systolic:diastolic ratio (AB ratio, S:D ratio impedance index)

$$= \frac{\text{systolic (max.)}}{\text{diastolic (min.)}}$$

In the umbilical artery all the vascular indices tend to decrease with advancing gestation and increasing compliance of the placenta (i.e. increased placental blood flow due to the decreased placental vascular resistance).

Absent End Diastolic Blood Flow Associations

- Normal in early pregnancy
- IUGR
- Premature delivery
- Oligohydramnios
- Toxemia of pregnancy
- Low Apgar score
- Increased incidence of fetal distress and need for cesarean section
- Increased ICU admission rate
- Increased risk of fetal death
- Systemic lupus erythematosus: absent or reversed diastolic flow velocity is detected in 11% pregnancies associated with SLE. This subgroup has an increased incidence of pre-eclampsia, IUGR, cesarian section and preterm delivery.

NB   Fetuses usually have acute or chronic hypoxia.

Discordant Umbilical Artery Flow Velocity

- Extensive placental infarction
- Retroplacental hematoma
- Discordantly sized umbilical arteries
- Spontaneous umbilical cord hematoma

Pulsatile Umbilical Venous Flow Late in First Trimester

- Normal fetuses: all pregnancies below 8 weeks gestation have a pulsatile flow, while none is evident in pregnancies beyond 13–15 weeks gestation. In normal second and third trimester fetuses pulsatile umbilical vein flow is absent only during fetal breathing

- IUGR/non-immune hydrops: considered a late and ominous sign of fetal compromise

- Abnormal karyotype: trisomy 13 and 18 but not in trisomy 21, monosomy X and triploidy.

Indications for Analysis of Fetal Umbilical Artery Waveforms

Suspected IUGR

Maternal hypertension and toxemia

Multiple gestation

In evaluation of twins, an abnormally high S:D ratio is frequently associated with IUGR (75%). In twin-twin transfusion syndrome the 'recipient' may have a lower S:D ratio than the donor twin.

Rhesus incompatibility

Placental abruption

Increased umbilical vein blood flow is found in placental abruption and may take some time to return to normal after antepartum hemorrhage has ceased.

Severe maternal illness

Hypertension

A reduction in diastolic flow velocity in the uteroplacental waveform has been reported. Hypertensive patients with normal utero-placental S:D ratios have a better fetal prognosis than those with abnormal waveforms.

Lupus anticoagulant syndrome

Abnormalities similar to those of toxemia of pregnancy have been reported. Abnormal uterine artery S:D ratios are indicative of patients at risk of IUGR and fetal death.

Sickle cell disease

Patients homozygous for sickle cell anemia have a high incidence of abnormal waveform ratios that correlate well with the presence of abnormal fetal cardiotocographs. The abnormalities are less prominent in the heterozygotes.

Maternal diabetes mellitus	There is a rise of umbilical vein volume flow rate, probably representing part of the fetal macrosomia syndrome.
Placenta previa	Placenta previa may cause an increase in the S:D ratio and those with high ratios (>3) have a significantly increased risk of perinatal mortality and morbidity. Umbilical vein blood flow may also be increased in placenta previa.
Oligohydramnios in post-term pregnancy	An elevated S:D ratio in the umbilical artery waveform is associated with increased fetal mortality and morbidity in gestations that are post term and have OH due to growth failure. There is no significant correlation in patients in whom the OH is secondary to rupture of membranes. Thus Doppler waveform is of limited value in post-term pregnancy at present.
Premature labor	Elevated S:D ratios in conjunction with uterine artery Doppler may indicate those at increased risk of premature delivery and thus aid management.
Congenital fetal abnormalities	Fetuses with cardiac abnormalities and abnormal flow waveforms have a poor prognosis particularly with absent end diastolic flow. Fetal death frequently occurs in this group. Doppler is helpful in assessing prognosis and thus planning management.

NB Reversed flow in the umbilical artery is associated with poor outcome.

Further Reading

Brown RN, Luzio LD, Gomes C & Nicolaides KH (1999) First trimester umbilical venous Doppler sonography in chromosomaly normal and abnormal fetuses. *J Ultra Med* 18: 543–546.

Challis DE, Warren PS & Gill RW (1995) The significance of high umbilical venous blood flow measurement in a high risk population. *J Ultrasound Med* 14: 907–912.

Favine D, Granovsky-Grisaru S, Ryan G et al (1998) Umbilical artery blood flow velocity in pregnancies complicated by systemic lupus erythematosus. *JCU* 26: 379–382.

Mires GT, Patel NV & Dempster J (1990) Review: The value of fetal umbilical artery flow velocity waveforms in the prediction of adverse fetal outcome in high risk pregnancies. *J Obstet Gynecol* 10: 261–270.

Sepulveda W, Shennan AH, Bowers S & Fisk NM (1995) Discordant umbilical artery waveforms in spontaneous umbilical cord hematoma. *JCU* 23: 330–332.

Thomas RL, Peng TCC, Eglinton GS et al (1991) Precision of umbilical artery Doppler studies. *J Ultrasound Med* 10: 201–204.

Vintzileos AM, Campbell WA & Rodis JF (1994) Antepartum assessment by ultrasonography. The fetal biophysical profile. In: Callen PW (ed.) *Ultrasonography in Obstetrics and Gynecology*, 3rd edn, pp 487–502, Philadelphia: WB Saunders.

Vascular Anomalies of the Umbilical Cord

Single umbilical artery	The cord usually has 3 vessels: 2 arteries and 1 vein surrounded by Wharton's jelly. An SUA is the most common umbilical cord anomaly with an incidence of 1% in singleton births and 46% in twin births. The prognosis is good in isolated anomaly. Congenital anomalies occur in 20% while cytogenetic anomalies are encountered in 17%. Trisomy 18, trisomy 13, Turner's and triploidy are associated in descending order of frequency. Most are diagnosed 2nd or 3rd trimester, there are a high number of false negatives before 20 weeks. SUA is related to primary agenesis or secondary atrophy; there is no familial tendency. In the absence of associated anomalies SUA on its own is not an indication for invasive karyotyping. US features: (1) The umbilical vein to umbilical artery diameter ratio of less than 2:1 is a good indicator of SUA; (2) transverse diameter >4 mm of umbilical artery between 20–36 weeks of gestation is a useful predictor of SUA; (3) abnormal systolic/diastolic ratio is an index of increased total peripheral resistance, which is usually associated with poor neonatal outcome; (4) color Doppler has further helped to diagnose SUA at an early gestational age.
Multivessel umbilical cord	This may be an antenatal indication of conjoined twinning.
Umbilical vein thrombosis	This is invariably related to fetal death.
Umbilical vein varix	See page 124.

Giant dilatation of the umbilical vein	This has been reported as causing a cystic fetal abdominal mass. The cyst showed slow moving particles within it, presumably due to turbulent blood flow and clot. Doppler/color evaluation shows flow.
Umbilical cord hemangioma	This may present as an umbilical cord mass. Doppler may be useful in diagnosis.
Umbilical cord knot, umbilical cord prolapse or nuchal cord	These are fetal life-threatening situations.
Persistent right umbilical vein (intrahepatic)	This is a rare finding: incidence 0.22%. The majority are not associated with any other anomalies. 28% are associated with lethal malformations. Sonographically best diagnosed on transverse sections to measure the abdominal circumference. The normal finding: left umbilical vein passes to the left of gallbladder and connects with the portal vein, it than curves right, away from the stomach. With the intrahepatic form of PRUV the umbilical vein passes lateral to the right side of the gallbladder joining the portal vein and curves towards the stomach. When the PRUV drains directly into the right atrium or into the IVC the aberrant vein runs anterior to the liver. Color flow Doppler facilitates identification of the abnormally placed venous pathway.
Absent ductus venosus	When the ductus venosus is absent the umbilical venous circulation drains into the portal vein or the systemic circulation – right atrium, IVC or iliac veins. Of the 16 cases reported in one series with absent ductus venosus with drainage into the systemic venous system none had a normal outcome, 7 had hydrops.

There are two umbilical veins in early gestation connecting the placenta to the embryo. They pass bilaterally outside the fetal liver through the splenic mesoderm - the septum transversum, between ipsilateral vitelline and common cardinal veins (sinus horns). There is gradual loss of bilateral symmetry affecting both sinus horns and their recipient veins. The first to go is the right umbilical vein usually at about the 4th week of gestation. Only the portion of the left umbilical vein closest to the sinus horn remains. The remaining part connects to the hepatic sinusoids. Anomalies of umbilical veins are rare.

NB   Color flow mapping and duplex Doppler are useful adjuncts to diagnosis in all the above conditions.

Anomalies Associated with a Single Umbilical Artery

Chromosomal anomaly (67%)

- Trisomy 18
- Trisomy 13
- Turners syndrome
- Triploidy

Cardiovascular (10%)

- VSD
- Conotruncal anomalies

Gastrointestinal (7.4%)

- Esophageal atresia

Central nervous system (4.7%)

- Hydrocephalus
- Holoprosencephaly
- Spina bifida

Genitourinary (3.18%)

- Hydronephrosis
- Dysplastic kidney

Respiratory (2.12%)

- Diaphragmatic hernia

Musculoskeletal (1.6%)

- Polydactyly
- Syndactyly

Abnormal cord insertions

- Marginal (18%)
- Velamentous (9%)

Head and neck

- Cystic hygroma
- Cleft lip

IUGR

Premature labor

Perinatal mortality (20%)

Stillbirth (66%)

Abdominal wall defects

Anomalies Associated with Persistent Umbilical Vein

Central nervous system

- Hydrocephaly
- Anencephaly
- Dandy-Walker syndrome
- Meningocele
- Ventriculomegaly
- Chiari II malformation

Cardiovascular system

- Mitral atresia
- Double outlet right ventricle
- Coarctation of aorta
- Asplenia
- ASD
- VSD
- Dextrocardia
- Total anomalous pulmonary venous drainage
- Hypertrophic cardiomyopathy
- Truncus arteriosus
- Aortic stenosis
- Atrial septum aneurysm

Urogenital

- Renal dysplasia
- Dysmorphic kidney
- Multicystic kidney
- Hypospadius
- Unicornuate uterus

Musculoskeletal

- Caudal regression
- Club feet
- Abnormal fibula
- Hemivertebra

Syndromes/multiple systems

- Noonan's syndrome
- IUGR
- Hydrops
- Fetal ascites
- Trisomy 18

Head and neck

- Nuchal folds
- Bilateral cleft lip

Most of the patients have been reported with multiple malformation.

Further Reading

Ariyuki Y, Hata T, Manabe A et al (1995) Antenatal diagnosis of persistent right umbilical vein. *JCU* 23: 324–326.

Catte LD, Osmanagasglu K & Schrijver ID (1998) Persistent right umbilical vein in trisomy 18: Sonographic observation. *J Ultra Med* 17: 775–779.

Cohen HL, Shapiro ML, Haller JO & Schwartz D (1992) The multisystem umbilical cord: an antenatal indicator of possible conjoined twinning. *JCU* 20: 278–282.

Estraff JA & Benacerraf BR (1992) Fetal umbilical vein varix: sonographic appearance and postnatal outcome. *J Ultrasound Med* 11:69–73.

Kirare AS, Ambardeker ST, Bhattacharya D & Pande SA (1996) Prenatal diagnosis with ultrasound of anomalous course of the umbilical vein and its relationship to fetal outcome. *J Clin Ultrasound* 24: 333–338.

Kirsch CFE, Feldstein VA, Goldstein RB & Filly RA (1996) Persistent intrahepatic right umbilical vein: A prenatal sonographic series without significant anomalies. *J Ultra Med* 15: 371–374.

Nyberg DA, Mahoney BS, Luthy D & Kapur R (1991) Single umbilical artery. Prenatal detection of concussed anomalies. *J Ultrasound Med* 10: 247–253.

Richards DS & Locksmith GJ (1998) Prenatal diagnosis of a bifurcating umbilical vein with left iliac vein connection. *J Ultra Med* 17: 185–189.

Vesce F, Huerrini P, Cavazzini L et al (1987) Ultrasonographic diagnosis of ectasia of the umbilical vein. *JCU* 15:346.

Wu M-H, Chong F-M, Shen M-R et al (1997) Prenatal sonographic diagnosis of a single umbilical artery. *JCU* 25: 425–430.

Causes of Umbilical Cord Masses

Cysts	Vitelline duct cysts Omphalomesenteric cyst Allantoic cyst Transient cyst – unknown etiology.
Umbilical cord hematoma	This may occur spontaneously (1:5500) or may follow cordiocentesis.
Accumulation of Wharton's jelly	This is usually of no pathological significance.
Hemangioma	Doppler ultrasound useful.
Teratoma	Rare tumor of the umbilical cord which may have cystic, solid or complex appearances on ultrasound.
Mucoid degeneration of the cord	
Knot in the umbilical cord	Usually a life-threatening situation.
Intrafetal umbilical vein varix	A varix of intrafetal umbilical vein is considered a poor prognostic sign; if no associated anomalies are present, the prognosis is generally good. Recently it has been suggested that this prenatal finding should be considered as a soft marker for aneuploidy (12%). Mortality associated with this anomaly has been reported between 24–44%. Differential diagnosis includes other abdominal cysts such as choledochal, mesenteric or urachal cysts. The presence of intra-abdominal umbilical vein varix can be confirmed by color Doppler finding of turbulent flow in the cystic mass.

Patent urachus

Ectasia of umbilical vein

Angiomyxoma   Solid or complex appearances on ultrasound.

Umbilical hernia   See page 266.

Further Reading

Estroff JA & Benacerraf BR (1992) Fetal umbilical vein varix: sonographic appearance and postnatal outcome. *J Ultrasound Med* 11: 69–73.

Fisk IJ & Filly RA (1989) Omphalocele associated with umbilical cord allantoic cysts: sonographic evaluation in utero. *Radiology* 149: 473.

Frazier HA, Guerrieri JP, Thomas RL et al (1992) The detection of patent urachus and allantoic cyst of the umbilical rod on prenatal ultrasonography. *J Ultrasound* 11(2): 117–120.

Jaunizux E, Moscoso G, Chitty L et al (1990) An angiomyxoma involving the whole length of the umbilical cord. *J Ultrasound Med* 9: 419.

Laccarino M, Baidi F, Perisco O et al (1986) Ultrasonic and pathologic study of mucoid degeneration of umbilical cord. *JCU* 14: 127.

Petrikovsky BM, Cooperman B, Kahn E & Pestrak H (1996) Prenatal diagnosis of non-iatrogenic hematoma of the umbilical cord. *JCU* 24: 37–39.

Causes of Umbilical Cord Enlargement

Maximum diameter = 1.76 cm at 32 weeks, the diameter reaches its plateau at 36 weeks gestation with a reduction in the Wharton's jelly content.

Fetal hydrops

Maternal diabetes	The cord diameter is significantly larger in fetuses of mothers with gestational diabetes and the main increase in the width is attributed to an increase in Wharton's jelly content.
Umbilical cord cysts	Both allantoic and omphalomesenteric cysts tend to occur close to the fetal end of the umbilical cord insertion. Incidental detection of umbilical cord cysts in early pregnancy is not associated with an adverse pregnancy outcome. A rare type of umbilical cord cyst is amniotic inclusion cyst (due to ectopic amniotic epithelium entrapped within the cord) which is usually an isolated abnormality.
Normal variant	Variation in the size of the umbilical vessels and amount of Wharton's jelly present.
Umbilical cord hematoma	The commonest cause of an umbilical cord hematoma is iatrogenic. Seventeen of the 36 cases of cord hematomas reported in the world literature resulted in fetal demise. Post-mortem examination of the cord in these cases revealed a venous source of bleeding. A solitary case of spontaneous cord hematoma in a viable fetus has been reported. Most hematomas result in fetal distress. US features a fusiform hyperechoic mass.
Umbilical cord tumors	Hemangioma and angiomyxofibroma, both are solid echogenic tumors; focal cord hematoma can give rise to a similar appearance.

Placental chorioangiomas	These tumors, when present on the placental surface, may involve the umbilical cord.
Mucoid degeneration	The umbilical cord is thickened (long segment) with cystic mass(es). The umbilical arterial velocimetry is normal. Antenatal diagnosis of mucoid degeneration of the umbilical cord has been reported with IUGR as well as normal fetal growth. Follow-up US scans showing normal fetal growth and normal umbilical Doppler velocimetry as well as reassuring fetal biophysical profile should allow continuation of pregnancy.

Reduced Wharton's Jelly

- Umbilical cord torsion
- IUGR
- Fetal distress during labor

Umbilical cord hematoma	1:5500 to 1:12 700 deliveries are associated with a cord hematoma with a fetal loss of 50%. US features include a hypoechoic mass, discordant umbilical artery Doppler waveforms in the absence of discordant umbilical arteries, ultrasonically normal placenta should raise the suspicion of compression of one umbilical artery.

Causes of umbilical cord hematoma

- Percutaneous umbilical blood sampling – most frequent cause
- Amniocentesis
- Torsion
- Traction
- Loops/knots (looping around fetal parts)
- Prolapse into an area of local weakness of Wharton's jelly
- Rarely spontaneous
- Short cord

Further Reading

Ami MB, Pertitz Y & Matilsky M (1999) Prenatal diagnosis of persistent right umbilical vein with varix. *JCU* 27: 273–275.

Casola G, Scheible W & Leopold GR (1985) Large umbilical cord: a normal finding in some fetuses. *Radiology* 156: 181.

Petrikovsky B, Gross B, Susin M & Holsten N (1995) Prenatal diagnosis of mucoid degeneration of the umbilical cord. *JCU* 23: 554–555.

Petrikovsky BM, Cooperman B, Kahn E & Pestrak H (1996) Prenatal diagnosis of non-iatrogenic hematoma of the umbilical cord. *JCU* 24: 37–39.

Sachs L, Fourcroj JL, Wenzel DJ & Nash JD (1982) Prenatal detection of umbilical cord allantoic cyst. *Radiology* 145:455.

Sepulveda W, Mackenna A, Sanchez J et al (1998) Fetal prognosis in varix of the intrafetal umbilical vein. *J Ultrasound Med* 17: 171–175.

Sepulveda W, Leible S, Ulloa A et al (1999) Clinical significance of first trimester umbilical cord cysts. *J Ultra Med* 18: 95–99.

Weissman A & Jakobi P (1997) Sonographic measurement of the umbilical cord in pregnancies complicated by gestational diabetes. *J Ultra Med* 16: 619–694.

Weissman A, Jacobi P, Bronstein M et al (1994) Sonographic measurements of umbilical cord and vessels during normal pregnancy. *J Ultra Med* 13: 11–14.

Ultrasound-Guided Intervention in Pregnancy

Amniocentesis (diagnosis)	*Indications* Early pregnancy – genetic: maternal age, previous chromosomal anomaly, balanced translocation, determine sex in sex-linked disorders, fetal anomalies with a high association with chromosomal abnormality. Inherited metabolic disorders – previous history/family history, racial group. Raised maternal AFP when no fetal abnormality detected and Finnish nephrosis suspected. Late pregnancy – to investigate extent of Rh isoimmunization, to determine fetal lung maturity, lecithin:sphingomyelin ratio and phosphatidylglycerol. *Risks* Fetal – fetomaternal hemorrhage, orthopedic deformities related to membrane rupture, increased risk of RDS, 1% chance of miscarriage/intrauterine death or preterm delivery. Fetal damage should be avoided by ultrasound guidance. Maternal – infection, amniotic leak; organ damage should be avoided by US guidance.
Amniocentesis for volume reduction in PH	To relieve maternal distress caused by PH and prevent or treat preterm labor. Placental abruption and rupture of membranes have been reported as complications.
Amniocentesis for pharmacologic intervention	Intra-amniotic drugs may be administered for cardiac arrhythmias (digitalis agents) or hypothyroid fetal goitre (thyroxine).

Chorionic villus sampling	First trimester alternative to amniocentesis performed between 10th and 12th weeks for cytogenetic, biochemical and molecular prenatal diagnoses.

Indications
Maternal age 35 or over. Previous offspring with chromosomal trisomy, parent carrier of chromosomal translocation, fetus at risk of an X-linked or metabolic/biochemical disorder. Screen positive on serum screening AFP/hCG. Abnormality on first trimester ultrasound associated with karyotypic abnormality.

Limitations
Transabdominal approach loss rate approximately 1.5–2.5% by experienced operators. Mosaicism from the placenta may necessitate fetal blood sample.

Percutaneous umbilical blood sampling	*Indications*

Blood group, hematocrit determination, transfusion, karyotyping (anomalies, severe IUGR), trans-placental infections, SLE, blood gas analysis in severe IUGR, hematological abnormalities, enzyme deficiency, blood chemistry (thyroxine in fetal goiter), hereditary immune deficiency and Duchenne's muscular dystrophy.

Complications
Fetal loss approx 1%. Cord hematoma and arterial spasm. Fetal movement can be abolished by pancuronium bromide.

Fetal transfusion/ intravascular therapy	Intravascular transfusion for anemia (Rh disease, severe anemia secondary to infection – parvo-virus). Intravascular drug therapy.

Fetal centesis and catheter placement	Abnormal fetal fluid collections may be aspirated for diagnostic or therapeutic reasons; fetal spaces can be decompressed into the amniotic cavity by a double pigtail catheter placement (bladder outflow obstruction, pleural effusions).
Selective termination	This may be performed in multiple pregnancy to selectively reduce fetal number, or to selectively terminate an abnormal fetus. Selective termination can be performed by ultrasound-guided intracardiac lethal injection of potassium chloride; 30% of patients lose the entire pregnancy.
Fetal biopsy	Skin and liver biopsy (congenital enzyme deficiency congenital ichthyosis). Rarely fetal tumors can be biopsied if the histology will alter obstetric management.

Further Reading

Copeland KL, Carpenter RJ, Fenolio KR & Ledbetter DH (1989) Integration of the transabdominal technique into an ongoing chorionic villus sampling program. *Am J Obstet Gynecol* 106: 1289-1294.

Evans MI, May M, Drugan A et al (1990) Selective termination: clinical experience and residual risks. *Am J Obstet Gynecol* 162: 1568-1575.

Finberg HJ & Clewell WH (1990) Ultrasound guided intervention in pregnancy. *Ultrasound* Q 3: 197-226.

Hobbins JC (1990) Chorionic villus sampling. In: Harrison MR, Golbus MS, Filly RA (eds) *The Unborn Patient*, pp 58-61. Philadelphia: WB Saunders.

Mahoney BS, Petty CN, Nyberg DA et al (1990) The stuck twin phenomenon: sonographic findings, pregnancy outcome and treatment with serial amniocentesis. *J Ultrasound Med* 9: 562.

Nicholaides KH, Soothill WP, Rodeck CW & Clewell WH (1986) Intravascular fetal blood transfusion by cordiocentesis. *Fetal Ther* 1: 185-192.

Perelman AH, Johnson RL, Clemons RD et al (1990) Intrauterine diagnosis and treatment of fetal goitrous hypothyroidism. *J Endocrinol Metab* 71: 618-621.

Social ML, MacGregor SN, Prelat BW et al (1987) Percutaneous umbilical blood transfusion in severe rhesus isoimmunization: resolution of fetal hydrops. *Am J Obstet Gynecol* 157: 1369-1374.

3

Structural Fetal Abnormalities

Screening for Chromosomal Abnormality

Age-related screening

There is a significant increase of chromosomal anomaly with advancing age, for example the risk of live-born Down's syndrome rises from 1 in 910 at aged 30 to 1 in 110 at aged 40. These data form the basis of invasive screening such as amniocenteses over a specific age group, usually 35 years old. However some data suggest that age-related screening is ineffective and results in only a 25% reduction in live-born Down's syndrome. Moreover if amniocentesis and karyotyping is restricted to women aged >35, 64–97% abnormal karyotype fetuses would be missed. When one considers the risk–benefit of amniocentesis the advantage gained is negated i.e. the risk of a Down's baby at age 37 is 1 in 240 while pregnancy loss as a result of amniocentesis is 1 in 200. A suggestion has been made that the risk of chromosomal anomaly is no higher at age >35, the increase in chromosomal anomaly simply reflects the fact that 13–14% of our mothers are aged 35 or over.

Biochemical screening

The sensitivity of biochemical screening using AFP is low at 21% but when combined with age-related screening the risk assessment can be improved. Low levels of serum AFP have been reported in Down's pregnancies varying between 0.63 and 1 MOM. The addition of other biochemical parameters such as measurement of human chorionic gonadotrophin and/or unconjugated estriol is said to improve detection but the results of the trials remain controversial.

Ultrasound screening

There are a number of major structural abnormalities detected on US with a clear association with chromosomal anomaly, such as omphalocele, but there are a multitude of so-called 'soft markers' with a controversial association. When two or more soft markers are detected the sensitivity for detection is improved. Sensitivity can be improved further by offering amniocentesis to mothers with major anomalies detected on US and targeted follow-up US to mothers with a single soft marker.

Sonographic Markers of Chromosomal Abnormalities

Central nervous system

- Ventriculomegaly
- Cerebellar dysplasia
- Holoprosencephaly
- Choroid plexus cysts – controversial risk from 0.75–9.5%*

Head and neck

- Nuchal translucency*
- Facial clefting*
- Abnormalities of head shape*
- Macroglossia*
- Micrognathia*
- Short ears*

Cardiac

- Atrioventricular septal defect
- Intracardiac echogenic foci*

Chest

- Pleural and pericardial effusions with and without hydrops
- Abnormality of breasts*

Gastrointestinal tract

- Omphalocele
- Intestinal obstruction
- Echogenic bowel*
- Cholecystomegaly*

Renal

- Hydronephrosis

Musculoskeletal

- Clindactyly, increased sandal gap*
- Shortening of long bones – femur and humerus*
- Abnormalities of iliac bones*

Umbilical cord abnormalities

- Single umbilical artery
- Umbilical cord cysts

Miscellaneous

- Abnormal amniotic fluid volume*

* Classed as 'soft markers.'

FETAL TRISOMIES AND SYNDROMES

Triploidy

Triploidy occurs when there are three sets of chromosomes instead of the two sets of diploidy (69 chromosomes). Severe IUGR associated with OH is the most prominent and consistent feature, other findings include abnormal head shape, cleft lip/palate, neural tube defects, CHD (ASD and VSD), hydrocephalus, holoprosencephaly, cystic renal dysplasia, club foot, syndactyly of fingers, omphalocele and large cystic placenta. The vast majority of fetuses with this phenotype abort spontaneously, usually in the first trimester. Twenty percent of all chromosomally abnormal abortuses are thought to be triploid.

Trisomy 21

(Down's syndrome) The most frequently occurring trisomy in liveborn. Sonographic features include: thickened nuchal skin fold (>3 mm in fetus 12–15 weeks), TOF, CHD (ASD, VSD, tetralogy of Fallot), duodenal atresia, hydrops fetalis, isolated pleural effusion/ascites, hypoplasia of the middle phalanx of the fifth finger (phalanges visible 15–16 weeks). There is increased sandal gap. The femoral and humeral lengths tend to be shorter than expected in relation to BPD. Currently less than 10% are detected antenatally. This may improve with careful screening, particularly cardiac. Intra-cardiac echogenic foci, which most probably represent microcalcification in the papillary muscles are present in 17% of Down's fetuses but only in 5% of normal fetuses. In a high-risk obstetric population the association between fetal intracardiac echogenic foci and trisomy 21 is said to be statistically significant. In the second trimester fetuses with trisomy 21 have greater iliac angle than fetuses with normal karyotype. The iliac angle varies with the axial level, the widest angle being at the most superior level. Measurement of the iliac angle should be taken at the most superior level. The frontal lobes of the cerebrum are statistically significantly smaller in Down's fetuses in the second trimester. US measurement of the frontothalamic distance (FTD) is a useful adjunct to diagnosis. FTD = inner table of frontal bone to the posterior margin of the thalamus. FTD is estimated from the estimated gestational age (EGA) with quadratic equation: $FTD = -0.0120 \times EGA^2 + 0.6917 \times EGA - 5.2349$ ($R^2 = 0.731$) or from the BPD with a linear equation: $FTD = 0.6837 \times BPD + 0.5525$ ($R^2 = 0.731$). If observed to expected ratio of 0.84 is used as a cut-off point to screen for Down's syndrome, a sensitivity of 16% and specificity of 97% are achieved.

Trisomy 18

(Edwards' syndrome) The second most common chromosomal anomaly. This is a lethal condition, most fetuses being lost perinatally. Sonographic features include IUGR, prominent occiput, PH or OH, micrognathia, low-set malformed ears, hydrocephalus, holoprosencephaly, myelomeningocele, choroid plexus cysts, short sternum, CHD (VSD, Fallot's tetralogy), diaphragmatic hernia, omphalocele, diaphragmatic hernia, polycystic kidneys, horseshoe kidney, PUJ obstruction, tracheoesophageal fistulas, hands held in abnormal position (clenched hand with overlapping index finger), talipes, shortened radial ray, clubbed forearm, clubbed foot, rocker-bottom foot.

Trisomy 13

(Patau's or Bartholin–Patau syndrome) Severe IUGR associated with PH, micro-ophthalmia, cleft lip/palate, polydactyly, digits held in fixed flexion, holoprosencephaly, omphalocele, CHD (90%), ACG, micrognathia, hypotelorism, malformed ears, hydronephrosis and polycystic kidneys. The condition is lethal.

Turner's syndrome | Sonographic features include a large cystic hygroma (70%) and hydrops, lymphangiectasia associated with hydrops fetalis, CHD (35%), coarctaion (15%), horse shoe kidney, skeletal abnormalities, including radial aplasia and symmetrical edema of the dorsum of feet. Cystic hygromas often regress.

Trisomy 9 | IUGR, craniofacial anomalies, misshapen ears, narrow chest, kyphoscoliosis, CHD, renal malformations, cystic dilatation of the fourth ventricle with lack of midline fusion. Prognosis is extremely poor.

Trisomy 20 | Craniofacial anomalies, hypo- or hypertelorism, large poorly formed ears, limb anomalies, vertebral defects, kyphoscoliosis, hydrocephalus, umbilical hernias, CHD and renal malformations. Prognosis depends upon associated malformations.

Trisomy 9P | Hypertelorism, prominent nose, cleft lip/palate, kyphoscoliosis and CHD; 10% die in early childhood, survivors have variable mental and other handicaps.

Trisomy 12 | Midface hypoplasia, small ears, turribrachycephaly with a high forehead, cleft palate, CHD and clindactyly of the 5th finger. Sonography is non-specific but when any combination of the above anomalies are seen, amniocentesis and chromosomal analysis are indicated.

Trisomy 10	IUGR, microcephaly, microphthalmia, cleft palate, malformed ears, camptodactyly, syndactyly, CHD, kyphoscoliosis, vertebral anomalies, brain and ocular malformations and gut malrotation; 50% die from CHD. Survivors are mentally retarded.
Trisomy 8	Prominent forehead, hypertelorism, camptodactyly of fingers and toes, hydrocephalus, CHD and urogenital anomalies; 10% die in the first 2 years. Mental retardation is mild to moderate.
Trisomy 10p	IUGR, dolichocephaly, dysplastic ears, cleft lip/palate, clubfoot, CHD and renal cystic disease. Half of the fetuses are stillborn or die in the postnatal period. Survivors show mental and motor deficiency.

ANOMALIES ASSOCIATED WITH TRISOMY 13

Central nervous system

- Holoprosencephaly (39%)
- Lateral ventricular dilatation
- Enlarged cisterna magna (58%)
- Microcephaly
- Posterior encephalocele
- Neural tube defects

Face and neck

- Cleft lip and palate
- Cyclopia
- Hypoplastic face
- Proboscis (48%)
- Hypotelorism
- Anophthalmia
- Nuchal thickening/cystic hygroma (21%)

Cardiac

- VSD
- Tetralogy of Fallot
- Hypoplastic left ventricle (48%)
- Transposition
- Echogenic chordae tendineae

The urinary tract

- Echogenic kidneys
- Enlarged kidneys (polycystic kidney) (33%)
- Hydronephrosis
- Horse-shoe kidney
- Bladder extrophy

Abdomen

- Echogenic bowel
- Omphalocele

Musculoskeletal

- Polydactyly
- Club/rocker bottom feet
- Clenched/overlying digits

Miscellaneous

- Severe IUGR
- Hydramnios
- Single umbilical artery

Drug Toxicity: Associated Malformations

Many drug-associated malformations are based on single or a few reports, which may be coincidental whilst other drugs are established teratogens marked with *.

IUGR

- Aspirin
- Busulfan
- Cocaine
- Cyclophosphamide
- Daunorubicin
- Ethanol*
- Heroin
- Lysergic acid diethylamide
- Marijuana
- Mechlorethamine
- Melphalan
- Mercaptopurine
- Methotrexate
- Oxazepam
- Paramethadione*
- Procarbazine
- Trimethadione*

Cardiac defects

- Amantadine
- Amobarbital
- Carbamazepine*
- Chlorambucil
- Chlordiazepoxide
- Clomiphene
- Coumarin derivatives
- Cystarabine
- Diphenhydramine
- Ethanol*
- Levothyroxine
- Lithium*
- Lysergic acid diethylamide
- Meclizine
- Norethynodrel

- Paramethadione*
- Procarbazine
- Prochlorperazine
- Quinine
- Retinoic acid*
- Sulfasalazine
- Tolbutamide
- Trimethadione*
- Valproic acid*

Musculoskeletal abnormalities

- Acetazolamide
- Aminopterin
- Para-amiosalicylic acid
- Amitryptyline
- Amobarbital
- Clomiphene
- Cocaine
- Coumarin derivatives
- Cyclophosphamide
- Cytarabine
- Diphenhydramine
- Disulfiram
- Ethanol*
- Etretinate*
- Fluorouracil
- Heroin
- Indomethacin
- Isoetharine
- Levothyroxine
- Lysergic acid diethylamide
- Mechlorethamine
- Meprobamate
- Methotrexate
- Metronidazole
- Nortriptyline
- Penicillamine
- Phenacetin
- Phenylephrine
- Phenytoin*
- Procarbazine
- Prochlorperazine

- Propoxyphene
- Quinine
- Retinoic acid*
- Sulfonamides
- Thioguanine
- Tolbutamide
- Trimethadione
- Quinine

Neural tube defects

- Aminopterin
- Carbamazepine*
- Etretinate*
- Norethindrone
- Oxazepam
- Quinine
- Valproic acid*

Microcephaly

- Chlordiazepoxide
- Chlorpromazine
- Chlorpropamide
- Chlomiphene
- Phenytoin*

Cleft lip/palate

- Aminopterin
- Amobarbital
- Busulfan
- Chlomiphene
- Coumarin derivatives
- Cyclophosphamide
- Diphenhydramine
- Fluphenazine
- Imipramine
- Mercaptopurine
- Phenytoin*
- Prochlorperazine
- Sulfasalazine
- Trimethadione
- Valproic acid*

Further Reading

Alfi OS & Lange M (1977) Trisomy 12p, a clinical recognisable syndrome. *Birth Defects* XIII(36): 231–232.

Anneren G, Fordis E & Jorcruf H (1981) Trisomy 8 syndrome. The rib anomaly and some new features in two cases. *Helv Paediatr Acta* 36: 465–472.

Benacerraf BR, Gelman R & Frigoletto D Jr (1987) Sonographic identification of second-trimester fetuses with Down's syndrome. *N Engl J Med* 317: 1371–1376.

Benacerraf BR, Osathanondh R & Frigoletto FD (1988) Sonographic demonstration of hypoplasia of the middle phalanx of the fifth digit: a finding associated with Down's syndrome. *Am J Obstet Gynecol* 159: 181–183.

Briggs GG, Freeman RK & Yaffe SJ (1990) *Drugs in Pregnancy and Lactation.* Baltimore, Williams & Wilkins.

Bundy AL, Saltzman DH, Pober B et al (1988) Antenatal sonographic findings in trisomy 18. *J Ultrasound Med* 5: 361–364.

Crane JP, Beaver HA & Cheung SW (1985) Antenatal ultrasound findings in fetal triploidy syndrome. *J Ultrasound Med* 4: 509.

Cullen MT, Green JJ, Scioscia AL et al (1995) Ultrasonography in the detection of aneuploidy in the first trimester. *J Ultrasound Med* 14: 559–563.

Dallapiccola B, Mastroiacovo PP, Montali E et al (1985) Trisomy 4p: five new observations and overview. *J Ultrasound Med* 4: 509.

De Vore GR (2000) Second trimester ultrasonography may identify 77–97% of fetuses with trisomy 18. *J Ultra Med* 19: 565–576.

Dubbins PA (1998) Screening for chromosomal abnormality. *Seminars in Ultrasound CT & MRI* 19: 310–317.

Edwards JH, Harnden DG, Cameron AH et al (1960) A new trisomic syndrome. *Lancet* I: 787–790.

Ginsberg J, Soukup S & Brendon RW (1989) Further observations of ocular pathology in trisomy 9. *Pediatr Ophthalmol Strabismus* 26: 146–149.

Hartley XY (1986) A summary of recent research into the development of children with Down's syndrome. *J Ment Defic Res* 30: 1–4.

Haslam R, Broske SP, Moor CM et al (1973) Trisomy 9 mosaicism with multiple congenital anomalies. *J Med Genet* 10: 180–184.

Hill LM, Guzick D, Belfor HL et al (1989) The current role of sonography in the detection of Down's syndrome. *Obstet Gynecol* 74: 620–623.

Jeanty P (1990) Prenatal detection of simian crease. *J Ultrasound Med* 9: 131–136.

Klep-de Poter JM, Billsman JB, de France HF et al (1979) Partial trisomy 10q. A recognisable syndrome. *Hum Genet* 46: 29–40.

Lehman CD, Nyberg DA, Winter TC, et al (1995) Trisomy 13: Prenatal US findings in a review of 33 cases. *Radiology* 194: 217–222.

Lockwood C, Scioscia A, Stiller R et al (1987) Sonographic features of triploid fetus. *Am J Obstet Gynecol* 157: 285.

Manning JE, Ragavendra N, Sayre J et al (1998) Significance of fetal intracardiac echogenic foci in relation to trisomy 21: A prospective sonographic study of high-risk pregnant women. *AJR* 170: 1083–1084.

Moerman P, Fryne KP, Goddeeris P et al (1987) Spectrum of clinical and autopsy findings in trisomy 18 syndrome. *Obstet Gynecol* 157: 285.

Morallo LM, Rosenblum H, Esterly KL et al (1983) Trisomy 18 (Edwards' syndrome) in Delaware. *Del Med J* 55(1): 27.

Nevin NC, Nevin J & Thompson W (1979) Trisomy 20. Mosaicism in amniotic fluid cell culture. *Clin Genet* 15: 440–443.

Pan SF, Fatona SR, Hoas JE et al (1975) Trisomy of chromosome 20. *Clin Genet* 9:445-453.

Patoo K, Smith DW, Therman E et al (1960) Multiple congenital anomalies caused by an extra autosome. *Lancet* I: 790-793.

Porreco RP, Matson MR, Young PE et al (1989) Diagnosis of a triploid fetus of genetic amniocentesis. *Obstet Gynecol* 56: 115.

Princan RA, Porto M, Towers CV et al (1989) Ultrasound findings in pregnancies complicated by fetal triploidy. *J Ultrasound Med* 8: 507-511.

Qazi QH, Hanachenapoomi R, Cooper R et al (1981) Duplication (12p) and (6) hypoplastic left heart. *Am J Med Genet* 9: 195-199.

Rethors MO, Larget-Piet L, Abony D et al (1970) Sur quatre cas de trisomie pour le bras court du chromosome 9. Individualisation d'une nouvelle entite morbide. *Ann Genet* 13: 217-232.

Sanchez JM, Fimtman N & Migliozine AM (1982) Report of a new case and clinical delineation of mosaic trisomy of a syndrome. *J Med Genet* 19: 384-386.

Shah YG, Eckl CJ, Stinson SK & Woods JR (1990) Biparietal diameter/femur length ratio, cephalic index and femur length measurements: not reliable screening techniques for Down's syndrome. *Obstet Gynecol* 75: 186-188.

Sheilds LE, Carpenter LA, Smith KM & Nghiem HV (1998) Ultrasonographic diagnosis of trisomy 18: Is it practical in the early second trimester. *J Ultra Med* 17: 327-331.

Smith DW (1982) *Recognisable Patterns of Human Malformation*. Philadelphia: WB Saunders.

Stabler GR, Buhler EM & Kleber JR (1963) Possible trisomy in chromosome group 6-12. *Lancet I*: 1379-1381.

Vergani P, Locatelli A, Piccoli MG et al (1999) Best second trimester sonographic markers for the detection of trisomy 21. *J Ultra Med* 18: 469-473.

Winter TC, Reichman JA, Luna JA (1998) Frontal lobe shortening in second trimester fetuses with trisomy 21: usefulness as an ultrasound marker. *Radiology* 207: 215-222.

Zook PD, Winter TC, Nyberg DA (1999) Iliac angle as marker for Down's syndrome in second trimester fetuses: CT measurement. *Radiology* 211: 447-451.

Fetal Skull and Neural Axis

Fetal Extracranial Masses

Encephalocele	The occiput is the most common site of the neural tube defect, which presents an echogenic appearance if brain substance is within the sac. Demonstration of a defect in the cranium is necessary to make a diagnosis. Ninety percent occur in the midline. May be purely cystic. There may be associated hydrocephalus and microcephaly.
Cystic hygroma	This is usually a neck mass and presents in the posterior nuchal region but the occiput may be affected. Sonography reveals a cystic mass with internal septations often associated with other anomalies.
Normal fetal hair	Hair around the fetal skull may occasionally be seen as bright scattered echoes which at times may mimic scalp edema or an encephalocele.
Hemangioma	Hemangioma can present in the occipital region but is usually more anterior in location. The sonographic appearance is one of homogeneous echogenic areas within a cystic mass. Doppler may be helpful.
Scalp edema	This is usually a part of a generalized anasarca related to the many causes of hydrops fetalis.
Teratoma	When this lesion presents in relation to the cranium it occupies a more anterior extracranial location, and sonographically is seen as an irregular mass with cystic and solid areas usually arising from the sphenoid and extending outward through the nasal and oral cavities. AFP is usually elevated.

Iniencephaly

This is an exceedingly rare anomaly, which affects the cranio-cervical junction manifesting itself as an extreme hyperextension of the cervical spine such that the occiput touches the spine. The anomaly is invariably associated with an occipital encephalocele and/or Dandy–Walker malformation. A crucial differential diagnosis is 'star-gazing breech' when the fetus assumes a position of extreme cervical hyperextension where there is usually no associated intracranial abnormality and the prognosis is good.

Further Reading

Bernstein HS, Filly RA, Goldberg JD & Globus MS (1991) Prognosis of fetuses with cystic hygroma. *Prenat Diagn* 11: 349–355.

Bromley B & Benacerraf BR (1995) The resolving nuchal fold in second trimester fetuses: not necessarily reassuring. *J Ultrasound Med* 14: 253–255.

Goldstein RB LaPidus AS & Filly RA (1991) Fetal cephaloceles: diagnosis with US. *Radiology* 180(3): 803–806.

Hanley ML, Guzman ER, Vintzileos AM et al (1996) Prenatal detection of regression of an encephalocele. *J Ultrasound Med* 15: 71–74.

Johnson MP, Johnson A, Holzgreve W et al (1993) First trimester simple hygroma: cause and outcome. *Am J Obstet Gynecol* 168(1 pt 1): 156–161.

Petrikovsky BM, Vintzileos AM & Rodis JF (1989) Sonographic appearance of occipital fetal hair. *JCU* 17: 425.

Rodis JF, Vintzileos AM, Campbell WA et al (1998) Spontaneous resolution of fetal cystic hygroma in Down's syndrome. *Obstet Gynecol* 71: 967–977.

Absence of Fetal Calvarium

Anencephaly	A common neural tube defect with a female preponderance of 4:1. Sonography reveals absence of brain and calvarium superior to the orbits. However, the appearance may be altered by the presence of rudimentary fibrovascular tissues superior to the orbits. These appear echogenic and may be quite sizeable in some fetuses. The cranial defect is symmetric in almost all cases. There is an associated polyhydramnios in the third trimester in 35% of cases.
Acrania	This is a rare anomaly distinct from anencephaly. There is partial or complete absence of the cranial vault. Brain tissue is always present but it may be abnormal. Thus the presence of brain tissue on sonography helps to differentiate from anencephaly.
Amniotic band syndrome	If the cranium is affected in amniotic band syndrome, the amputation defect is invariably asymmetric. Other fetal parts may be involved, e.g, limbs, body wall, spine, etc. The amniotic band may be visible sonographically.
Severe microcephaly	Microcephaly, when severe, may mimic anencephaly; however, one can always identify a cranial vault and frequently cortical brain tissue. With anencephaly both the vault and brain tissue are missing.
Exencephaly and cranioschisis	Large amount of disorganized cerebral tissue arising from the base of the skull but the calvarium is absent. The facial structures are preserved. Exencephaly is regarded as an embryonic precursor of anencephaly, an anomaly incompatible with life.

Holoacardious acephalic twin

This is a rare occurrence and can represent a true anencephalic anomaly. The entire cranium may be lacking or there may be severe microcephaly. This condition occurs only in identical twins.

Poorly mineralized cranium

Defective bone mineralization in conditions such as osteogenesis imperfecta and congenital hypophosphatasia may result in poor definition of the cranial vault on sonography. Careful scanning almost always shows a thin but deformed calvarium with normal underlying brain tissue.

Further Reading

Bromley B & Benacerraf BR (1995) Difficulties in the prenatal diagnosis of microcephaly. *J Ultrasound Med* 14: 303–305.

Filly RA (1994) In: Callen PW (ed.) *Ultrasonography in Obstetrics and Gynecology*, 3rd edn, pp 189–234. Philadelphia: WB Saunders.

Goldstein RB & Filly RA (1988) Prenatal diagnosis of anencephaly. Spectrum of sonographic appearances and distinction from amniotic band syndrome. *AJR* 151: 247–250.

Hautman GD, Sherman SJ, Utter GO et al (1995) Acrania. *J Ultrasound Med* 14: 552–554.

Hendricks SK, Cyr DR, Nyberg DA et al (1998) Exancephaly: clinical and ultrasonic correlation. *Obstetrics & Gynaecology* 72: 898.

Mahoney BS, Filly RA, Callen PW & Golbus MS (1985) The amniotic band syndrome: antenatal sonographic diagnosis and potential pitfalls. *Am J Obstet Gynecol* 152: 63.

Patel MD, Swinford AE & Filly RA (1994) Anatomic and sonographic features of the fetal skull. *J Ultrasound Med* 13(4): 251–257.

Tongsong T, Sirichotiyakul S & Siriangkul S (1995) Prenatal diagnosis of congenital hypophosphatasia. *JCU* 23: 52–55.

Small Fetal Cranium

Wrong dates

With good menstrual history this problem is unlikely to arise; however, difficulty may occur in women with irregular menstrual periods or ovulation induction. When in doubt, serial ultrasonic scans with BPD, head circumference and cephalic index measurements may resolve the issue.

IUGR

Fetuses suffering from IUGR are small for dates. IUGR may be symmetrical or asymmetrical. Symmetrical IUGR occurs as a result of severe insult in early pregnancy. The fetus is symmetrically small. There is a proportionate reduction in all body parts. This form of IUGR can be diagnosed on ultrasound if accurate dates are unknown, preferably by CRL measurement.

Microcephaly

Microcephaly is associated with a multitude of syndromes, chromosomal anomalies, transplacental infections and maternal addictions. It may also be inherited in an autosomal recessive manner. Diagnosis can be difficult as microcephaly may not develop until late in pregnancy. Prenatal diagnosis is not excluded by normal biometry on second trimester US.

Further Reading

Bromley B & Benacerraf BR (1995). Difficulties in the prenatal diagnosis of microcephaly. *J Ultrasound Med* 14: 303-305.

Fetal Disorders Associated with Microcephaly

Cornelia De Lange syndrome

Autosomal dominant but can be sporadic, characterized by IUGR microcephaly, brachycephaly, micrognathia, micromelia, syndactyly and cardiac defects.

Freeman Sheldon syndrome

(Whistling face syndrome) Autosomal dominant but cases are sporadic, characterized IUGR, abnormal facies with sloping forehead, deep set eyes, small nose; microcephaly, ulnar deviation of hands, clubbed feet, and contractures of hips and knees.

Neu Laxova syndrome

Autosomal recessive characterized by IUGR, severe microcephaly, receding forehead, cleft lip/palate, micrognathia, flat nose, proptosis, cataracts, absent eyelids, cystic hygroma, hypertelorism, short neck, hypodentia, lissencephaly, dysgenesis of the corpus callosum, hypoplasia of cerebellum, Dandy–Walker anomaly, limb contractures, rocker bottom feet, kyphosis, skin syndactyly, hypoechoic skeleton, skin syndactyly, swelling of knees and elbow joints, unilateral renal agenesis, curved penis, cryptorchidism, ichthyosis, pulmonary hypoplasia, CHD, feeble cardiac activity, PH, short umbilical cord, edema of scalp, edema of hands and feet and small placenta.

Miller Dieker syndrome

(Lissencephaly type 1) Deletion at 17p13.3 locus, those with balanced translocation at risk of bearing offspring with this disorder, characterized by lissencephaly, microcephaly (late onset), mid-ventriculomegaly, IUGR and cardiac defects.

Rubella syndrome

This occurs as a result of rubella virus infection before eight weeks gestation. The syndrome is characterized by IUGR, CHD, eye defects, microcephaly, and hepatosplenomegaly.

Seckel syndrome

Autosomal recessive disorder characterized by early onset IUGR, microcephaly, severe micrognathia, prominent nose, flexion deformity of hips and knees.

Smith–Lemli–Opitz

Autosomal recessive, characterized by microcephaly, genital abnormalities, syndactyly, post axial polydactyly, clenched hands, hydronephrosis, renal hypoplasia, cystic kidneys, nuchal lucency in first trimester and late-onset IUGR.

Toxoplasmosis

This is the result of intrauterine infection with *Toxoplasmosis gondii.* The syndrome is characterized by IUGR, microcephaly, ventriculomegaly, intracranial calcifications, cataracts, hepatic calcifications, hepatomegaly, increased AC, ascites and thickened placenta.

Varicella

First or second trimester infection with varicella virus characterized by ventriculomegaly, microcephaly, clubbed feet, abnormally positioned hands, hepatomegaly, two vessel cord, hydrops and PH.

Spina Bifida

Arnold–Chiari	Between 80 and 90% seen as an abnormal banana-shaped cerebellum or absent cerebellum.
Ventriculomegaly	75% of cases of spina bifida demonstrate this abnormality.
Lemon-shaped head	Seen in 90–95% of fetuses with spina bifida.
Abnormal spine	The majority (63%) occur in the lumbosacral region where the abnormally wide and divergent lateral masses are evident. There may be skin covering or just a thin membrane. Open – 80%; closed – 20%.
Open spina bifida	13% are associated with aneuploid fetuses; the likelihood of an associated anatomic abnormality has been found in 40% although in one study only 22% of these were detectable on US. If the spina bifida is an isolated abnormality on US a 4% chance of aneuploidy still persists. Prenatal US can help to predict karyotypically abnormal fetuses with spina bifida but 20% will be missed if US is used alone in the setting of a prenatally detected spina bifida. Some authors believe that cytogenetic analysis is justified in these instances.
Bifid sacrum artifact	A bifid sacrum artifact is a skewed representation of normal anatomy and should not be interpreted as a true anomaly. It is produced by a steeply angled parasagittal scanning plane that intersects normal structures. Sonograms of the distal fetal spine can be misleading and deceptive. The normal spine is constructed of multifaceted anatomic structures that change in appearance and relative position throughout gestation. These complex structures can be seriously misinterpreted if scanning planes are skewed or rotated off axis.

Further Reading

Babcook CJ, Goldstein RB & Filly RA (1995) Prenatally detected fetal myelomeningocele: Is karyotype analysis warranted? *Radiology* 194: 491–494.

Babcook CJ, Ball RH & Feldkamp ML (2000) Prevalence of aneuploidy and additional anatomic abnormalities in fetuses with open spina bifida: population based study in Utah. *J Ultra Med* 19: 619–623.

Kliewer MA, Hertzberg BS, George P et al (1995) Fetal bifid sacrum artifact: developmental anatomy simulating malformation. *Radiology* 195: 673–676.

Nicolaides KH, Campbell S & Gabbe SG (1986) Ultrasound screening for spina bifida: cranial and cerebellar signs. *Lancet* ii: 72–74.

Wormian Bones

Wormian bones are small irregular ossicles located within the cranial sutures, 50% occur within the lambdoid sutures and about a quarter are located within the coronal sutures. Although they may occur as a normal anatomical variant, there is a large body of literature which describes an association with congenital anomalies. In one study (Pryles & Khan, 1979) the prevalence of CNS anomalies in a population with Wormian bones varied from 93% to a 100% in a random group and reached a 100% in a mentally retarded population. A variety of non-CNS anomalies have been reported (see gamut). When they occur as normal variant they are smaller and less numerous. A variant of Wormian bones is the partial Wormian bones – a peninsular formation, in which the Wormian bones are partially attached to normal cranium. Sonographically Wormian bones appear as well circumscribed islands of tissue of bone echogenicity within the fontanelles. A tangential section of the skull at the level of the posterior fontanelle allows diagnosis to be made.

Wormian bones: associated anomalies

Common

- CNS anomalies (including craniostenosis, microcephaly, macrocephaly, hydrocephalus and dysgenesis of corpus callosum)

- Normal variant
  Isolated low set ears
  Single umbilical artery
  Congenital heart disease
  Cleidocranial dysplasia
  Osteogenesis imperfecta
  Hypophosphatasia
  Hypothyroidism
  Pyknodysostosis
  Tracheomalacia (congenital)

Rare

- Trisomy 21
- Chondrodysplasia punctata
- Hallerman-Streiff syndrome
- Oto-palato-digital syndrome
- Metaphyseal chondrodysplasia (Jansen)
- Aminopterin fetopathy
- Menkes syndrome (kinky hair syndrome)
- Hajdu–Cheney syndrome
- Osteopetrosis (infantile)
- Zellweger syndrome
- Idiopathic familial osteoarthropathy
- Grant syndrome
- Sclerosteosis
- Mandibuloacral dysplasia
- Aplasia cutis congenita
- Congenital cutis laxa

Further Reading

Pryles CV & Khan AJ (1979) Wormian bones: A marker for CNS abnormality? *Am J Dis Child* 133: 380.

Jeanty P, Silva SR & Turner C (2000) Prenatal diagnosis of Wormian bones. *J Ultra Med* 19: 863–869.

Fetal Ventriculomegaly

Obstructive hydrocephalus – etiology

Spina bifida

Spina bifida may occur at any location along the spine but is most common in the lumbosacral region. Spina bifida is diagnosed when the posterior ossification centers splay outwardly and are further apart than the ossification centers above or below the defect. The cleft in the soft tissues is usually easily identified when the sac is intact and bulges into the amniotic cavity but findings can be minimal or absent. Spina bifida accounts for approximately 30% of all cases of ventriculomegaly. Sonographic examination of the head may demonstrate the 'lemon' and 'banana' signs. The 'banana' sign is related to the cerebellum when it is curved around the mid-brain to produce a banana-shaped structure. The lemon is the abnormal cranial shape. Associated anomalies involving other organs are common in spina bifida.

Dandy–Walker malformation

This syndrome is usually the result of abnormal development of the cerebellum and fourth ventricle. The fourth ventricle is seen as an enlarged cystic structure in the posterior fossa with splaying of the cerebellar hemispheres. The cerebellar vermis usually shows hypoplasia. Hydrocephalus is seen in up to 70% of fetuses. Associated anomalies involving other organs are fairly common. Prognosis depends on associated chromosomal anomalies and other organ defects.

Artifact

Apparent ventriculomegaly may be recorded if an oblique view is inadvertently used to image the ventricle.

Cranial Cavity Mainly Fluid – Filled

Alobar holoprosencephaly

This condition is produced when the two cerebral hemispheres fail to divide. Alobar type is the most severe form with a monoventricle, a dorsal sac of varying size and fused thalami. The falx, corpus callosum, optic and olfactory tracts are absent. The midbrain, brainstem and cerebellum usually appear normal. The presence of anterior cerebral cortex and hippocampal ridge differentiates this condition from hydranencephaly. The head in the alobar type is usually small. Identification of cavum septum pellucidum excludes the diagnosis of holoprosencephaly of all types. Associated anomalies, particularly of the face, are common.

Hydranencephaly

Hydranencephaly is seen as a large monoventricular cystic structure within the fetal cranium with no cerebral cortex. The falx is usually present but the thalami absent. The condition represents a destructive brain process, most probably as a result of an in-utero vascular accident. The choroid plexus may be preserved so that the head may be small, but with a functioning choroid plexus hydrocephalus may develop. There are normally no associated anomalies but the prognosis is poor.

Aqueduct stenosis

This is related to narrowing of the aqueduct which may be secondary to inflammation, maldevelopment or rarely inherited in X-linked manner. There is enlargement of both lateral and third ventricles. The fourth ventricle and cerebellum are usually normal.

Spinal dysraphism — This refers to abnormal or incomplete fusion of the midline dorsal region during embryogenesis. It may be divided into two groups: the open form includes an intracanalicular lipoma, diastematomyelia (presenting as a central bright linear echo within the spinal canal of a widened level) and a tethered cord. Ventriculomegaly is often associated.

Meckel's syndrome — This is an autosomal recessive disorder associated with a posterior encephalocele, hydrocephalus, there is microcephaly secondary to cerebral and cerebellar hypoplasia (small head diameter), large kidneys due to bilateral non-obstructive dysplasia, empty bladder and OH. Other variable features include facial clefts, sloped forehead, CHD and pulmonary hypoplasia.

Choroid plexus papilloma — These are small benign tumors which arise from the normal choroid plexus. They are echogenic masses and can be differentiated from blood clot by their pulsating vascularity. They may cause hydrocephalus; sonography may reveal a mass within a dilated ventricle.

Cloverleaf skull deformity — The term kleeblattschadel means 'with cloverleaf'. The cloverleaf skull is an enlarged trilobed head deformity which results from premature fusion of the coronal and lambdoid sutures, associated with hydrocephalus. The anomaly is subdivided into type I (the more severe form associated with thanatophoric dysplasia) and type II (associated with less severe skeletal abnormalities). Type III is an isolated anomaly with the best prognosis. Differential diagnosis is from craniostenosis, ABS and Apert's syndrome (congenital craniostenosis and syndactyly of hands and feet, associated visceral malformation include dextrocardia and pyloric stenosis).

Arachnoid cysts

Most arachnoid cysts are acquired. Congenital cysts are extremely rare. These cysts produce a mass effect within the fetal cranium and may result in hydrocephalus. Arachnoid cysts must be distinguished from other supratentorial cysts.

Intracranial bleed

These occur in the third trimester and result in secondary obstruction at the adequate level.

Non-Obstructive Ventriculomegaly

Agenesis of corpus callosum

Dysgenesis of the corpus callosum ranges from complete to partial absence and may be detectable on ultrasound in utero from about 17 weeks onwards. Standard second trimester US before 22 weeks may not show isolated ACC. Fetuses with this abnormality can have normal second-trimester scans and develop abnormal US findings in the third trimester. On a midline sagittal US the corpus callosum forms a broad-arched echo-poor band in the floor of the intrahemispheric fissure. It is delineated superiorly by echogenic pericallosal cisterns and the inferior surface forms the roof of cava septi pellucidi and frontal horns of the lateral ventricle. Secondary abnormalities of the ventricles and cerebral hemispheres are the key to the diagnosis of ACC. The ventriculomegaly associated with ACC, termed 'colpocephaly' is due to poor development of the cerebral cortex. The ventriculomegaly in ACC is much more pronounced in the occipital horns. The cavum septum is absent, the lateral ventricles are placed wide apart with both the lateral and medial walls aligned more parallel to the midline. There may be concave configuration of the medial ventricular wall due to protrusion of the cingulate gyrus and uncrossed white matter tracts (i.e. bundles of Probst). The third ventricle is dilated and may herniate upwards between the two displaced lateral ventricles. There is a radial arrangement of medial cerebral sulci. Associated anomalies include trisomy 13 and 18, DWM and holoprosencephaly.

Colpocephaly

This condition is often associated with agenesis of the corpus callosum or holoprosencephaly and is the term applied to ventriculomegaly due to inadequate development of the cerebral cortex. The pressure within the ventricles is normal.

Holoprosencephaly

Holoprosencephaly is produced with non-development of the two cerebral hemispheres and ventricles. It is subdivided into three types: alobar, semilobar and lobar. Alobar is the most severe (see page 159). In the semilobar type sonography reveals a mono-ventricle with rudimentary occipital horns which connect with the dorsal sac. The thalami are usually partially fused. The lobar type is the mildest type with partial division of the lateral ventricle, fused anterior horns but fairly well separated occipital horns. The head size may be enlarged, small or normal. Associated anomalies are common, including chromosomal.

Hydranencephaly

There is no discernible cerebral cortex. The most striking sonographic feature is an almost fluid-filled cranium with a 'monoventricle.' The falx is usually present but the thalami are absent. The condition is not inherited and has no associated anomalies.

Fryns syndrome

Autosomal recessive disorder characterized by dysmorphic features, diaphragmatic hernia, distal limb hypoplasia, pulmonary hypoplasia and multiple CNS, GIT and genitourinary abnormalities. Initially thought to be lethal but recent reports of survival through the neonatal period with severe developmental delay. US features include diaphragmatic hernia, cleft lip/palate, ACC and ventriculomegaly, gastric anomalies, bilateral renal enlargement, cystic hygroma, fetal hydrops and PH.

Further Reading

Agapitos E & Christodoulou C (1995) Meckel–Gruber syndrome associated with Rokitansky–Kuster–Hauser syndrome. *JCU* 23: 452–455.

Brocard D, Regag C, Vibert M et al (1993) Prenatal diagnosis of X-linked hydrocephalus. *JCU* 21: 211–214.

Filly RA & Goldstein RB (1994) Fetal ventricular atresia: fourth down and 10 mm to go. *Radiology* 193: 315.

Gembruch U, Baschat AA, Reusche E et al (1995) Fetal aqueduct stenosis diagnosed sonographically: how grave is the prognosis? *AJR* 164: 725–726.

Patel MD, Filly AL, Hersh DR & Goldstein RB (1994) Isolated fetal cerebral ventriculomegaly: clinical course and outcome. *Radiology* 192(3): 759–764.

Twinning D, Jaspar T & Zuccollo J (1994) Outcome of fetal ventriculomegaly. *Br J Radiol* 67(793): 26–31.

Bennett GL, Bromley B & Benacerraf BR (1996) Agenesis of corpus callosum: prenatal detection usually is not possible before 22 weeks of gestation. *Radiology* 199: 447–450.

Sheffield JS, Twickler DM Timmons C et al (1998) Fryns syndrome: prenatal diagnosis and pathologic correlation. *J Ultra Med* 17: 585–589.

Differential Diagnosis of Fetal Intracranial 'Cyst'

Large cisterna magna	The cisterna magna lies between the cerebellum and the occipital bone, with a normal AP diameter of 4–10 mm. A cisterna magna larger than 10 mm suggests Dandy–Walker malformation. Other associations include communicating hydrocephalus, cerebellar hypoplasia and retrocerebellar arachnoid cyst. Cisterna magna >10 mm in AP diameter on its own is not a significant finding, however a detailed examination should be undertaken but if the fetus is normal neither karyotype testing nor postnatal neurological evaluation is needed.
Non-obstructive hydrocephalus	Ventriculomegaly means dilatation of the ventricles, which may be obstructive (hydrocephalus) or non-obstructive. These are difficult to differentiate antenatally. The non-obstructive variety may be associated with agenesis of the callosum, which shows mildly dilated lateral ventricles, absent falx and normal thalami. Dandy–Walker malformation, alobar holoprosencephaly and hydranencephaly are other conditions associated with non-obstructive ventriculomegaly.
Obstructive hydrocephalus	Since it is difficult to determine intraventricular pressure safely in the fetus, obstructive hydrocephalus should not be diagnosed in utero unless an enlarging head and ventricles are documented on serial scans. The majority of cases of obstructive hydrocephalus in the fetus are due to aqueduct stenosis. In this instance there is dilatation of the lateral and third ventricles. A normal BPD or head circumference does not exclude hydrocephalus.

Choroid plexus

CPCs are common. They usually disappear by 26 weeks. Cysts persisting longer should be considered of different origin. They may be multilocular, varying in size from 3 to 13 mm. They have been reported in association with anomalies, which include trisomies 21 and 18, Goldenhar's syndrome, agenesis of the corpus callosum, frontal lipomas, frontal meningoceles, median cleft nose, hypertelorism, cervical spinal anomalies and cardiac defects.

'Midline cyst' in ACC

In agenesis of the corpus callosum the third ventricle may enlarge dramatically and herniate upwards, sandwiched between the two hemispheres. This produces the so-called midline or 'interhemispheric cysts.'

Holoprosencephaly

This is related to failure of the brain to divide into two hemispheres and two ventricles. This results in a monoventricle with an absent falx and fused midline thalami. Other associated anomalies include trisomies 13 and 18, triploidy, omphalocele and renal dysplasia. Facial abnormalities such as cyclopia, midline clefting and hypotelorism are usually associated.

The alobar type is the most severe brain abnormality. The midbrain, brainstem and cerebellum are normal. The corpus callosum, fornix, falx cerebri, optic tracts and olfactory bulbs are absent. The cerebral cortex is small, lies anteriorly and forms a 'horse-shoe' shape. The dorsal cyst has no cortical mantle.

Arachnoid cysts	These are either abnormalities of development of the leptomeninges or secondary to hemorrhage or infection. These cysts may produce a mass effect and secondary hydrocephalus.
Schizencephaly	This term is applied to bilateral clefts in the cerebral cortex in the region of the middle cerebral arteries. Sonography reveals fluid collections which communicate with the lateral ventricles bilaterally and extend to the calvarium.
Porencephaly	Porencephaly results from infarction or hemorrhage into the brain, necrosis follows. The necrotic brain parenchyma may evacuate into the ventricular cavity or subarachnoid space. The result is a cyst in free communication with the ventricle or a subarachnoid cistern. The porencephalic cyst does not produce a mass effect.
Posterior fossa arachnoid	A retrocerebellar arachnoid cyst is a less common and more benign abnormality than the Dandy–Walker malformation. The cyst may produce a mass effect, displacing the hemispheres.
Cystic periventricular leukomalacia	CPL usually appears as cystic structures adjacent to the angle of the frontal horns. The cysts vary from 2 to 5 mm. Although the diagnosis has been made antenatally, it is often not diagnosed due to the relatively low position of the fetal head in the pelvis making imaging of the cortical region difficult late in pregnancy. It has a significant association with handicap.

Vein of Galen aneurysm	Vein of Galen aneurysms are basically arterio-venous malformations. The venous limb is represented by cystic dilatation of the vein of Galen. They are rare lesions. The cystic dilatation of the vein of Galen is supratentorial in location, in communication with tubular vessels leading to and from it. Turbulent high-frequency Doppler signals are obtained. There may be secondary hydrocephalus or high-output failure secondary to a large AV shunt.
Subdural collections	Rarely seen antenatally, usually occurs secondary to a fetal bleeding diathesis.
Unilateral hydrocephalus	Unilateral hydrocephalus is rare, ventriculo-megaly is therefore assumed to be bilateral and symmetric even if the near-field ventricle is obscured by artifact. The causes include agenesis/stenosis of the foramen of Monro, transient obstruction of the foramen, intra-ventricular hematoma and underlying brain dysplasia. Prognosis is usually favorable. True unilateral ventricular dilatation may be seen in megaloencephaly – a migration disorder.
In-utero cerebral hemorrhage	Classified into four types: type I confined to the germinal matrix; type II subependymal hemor-rhage with rupture into the ventricle; type III same as II but with ventricular dilatation; type IV extension of hemorrhage into the brain parenchyma. All cases diagnosed in utero have been type III or IV. Intraparenchymal hemor-rhage may show progressive liquefaction, which eventually results in a porencephalic cyst. The associated hydrocephalus secondary to aqueduct stenosis may be progressive.

NB US assessment of the width of the lateral ventricular atrium is valuable in detection of fetal ventriculomegaly, which is the most sensitive sonographic indicator of maldevelopment of the fetal brain and spinal cord. The atrial diameter is used to determine the normality of ventricular size. The atrial diameter has been shown to have a stable width throughout the gestational period with a mean atrial diameter of 6.5 mm and a standard deviation of 1.3. Many use 10 mm as the upper limit for a normal atrial size but when the atrial diameter exceeds 10 mm, a detailed examination of the fetus is undertaken. In some fetuses with atrial diameter over 10 mm no other abnormality is detectable on US, which has been termed 'isolated mid ventriculomegaly' (IMV). Although some of the fetuses with IMV later prove to have co-existing abnormalities that have been missed on a prenatal US. However the majority of fetuses develop normally. Male fetuses have a slightly larger atrial size than female fetuses. Female fetuses have a mean atrial diameter of 5.8 ± 1.3 mm (SD) and male fetuses 6.4 ± 1.3 mm (SD). The choroid usually fills the atrial lumen. If fluid is seen between the choroid and the ventricular wall, measurement becomes necessary.

Altered Third Ventricular Morphology

At any gestational age a third ventricle >3.5 mm in width should be regarded as abnormal. The width of the 3rd ventricle is relatively stable at approximately 1 mm in the second and early third trimester. After 32 weeks the width increases to 2 mm.

Hydrocephalus	The dilated third ventricle splays the anterior the anterior portion of the thalami.
Holoprosencephaly	The third ventricle is absent and the thalami fused.
Agenesis corpus callosum	Enlarged and high riding, may extend superior to the level of the thalami as an inter-hemispheric 'cyst'.
Space-occupying lesions	Colloid cyst or choroid plexus papilloma may enlarge the third ventricle.
Cavum septum pellucidum	This is a normal anatomic structure and should not be confused with the third ventricle.

Midline Cystic Brain Lesions

Cavum velum interpositum	V-shaped cystic structure pointing anteriorly.
Arachnoid cyst of velum interpositum	
AV malformation of velum interpositum	
Aneurysm of vein of Galen	High-frequency turbulent waveforms on spectral Doppler that fill with color.
Interhemispheric cyst associated with ACC	Cyst extends cephalad between cerebral hemispheres or when dysmorphic features of ACC – such as colpocephaly or radiating gyral pattern.
Dilated third ventricle	
Suprasellar arachnoid cyst	More rounded located more anteriorly than the cyst of the velum interpositum.

Anomalies Associated with Agenesis of Corpus Callosum

Central nervous system anomalies

- Hydrocephalus
- Midline intracerebral lipoma
- Interhemispheric cyst
- Arnold–Chiari II malformation
- Holoprosencephaly
- Porencephaly
- Encephalocele
- Median cleft syndrome
- Lissencephaly II (muscle-eye-brain disease; cerebro-oculo-muscular syndrome)
- Gray-matter heterotopia

Chromosomal disorders

- Trisomies 18, 13 and 15

Non-chromosomal syndromes

- Acrocallosal syndrome – probably autosomal recessive, rare associated with ACC, micropolgyria, Dandy–Walker malformation and limb anomalies
- Andermann syndrome, autosomal recessive, the majority of cases reported from the Province of Quebec, Canada, associated with partial or complete ACC
- Apert syndrome – sporadic cases, some autosomal dominant transmission. A variety of malformations are reported but prenatal US diagnosis is dependent on demonstration of acrocephaly, cupped hands; fusion of digits
- Fetal alcohol syndrome (see page 199)
- Frontonasal syndrome (see page 210)

- Joubert syndrome – autosomal recessive, present with hyperventilation and apnea, hypotonia, peculiar eye movements with delayed motor milestones in neonatal period. There are a variety of CNS, eye, liver and renal abnormalities. Antenatal diagnosis is based on the demonstration of hypoplasia of cerebellar vermis, ACC and large cisterna magna communicating with a dilated fourth ventricle
- Neu–Laxova syndrome (see page 203)
- Oro-facial-digital 1 syndrome – X-linked dominant inheritance, lethal in males characterized by facial and CNS anomalies including hypertelorism, median cleft lip, microcephaly, encephalocele, ACC, hydrocephalus and several hand and digital abnormalities. Polycystic kidneys have also been reported
- Rubenstein–Taybi syndrome – sporadic, a few familial cases have been reported, a multitude of multisystem abnormalities have been reported besides many facial anomalies and ACC
- Shapiro syndrome/reverse Shapiro syndrome – exceptionally rare syndrome with mostly functional abnormalities, the only anatomical abnormality reported is ACC associated with periodic hyperthermia

Further Reading

Benacerraf BR (1987) Asymptomatic cysts of the fetal choroid ± plexus in the second trimester. *J Ultrasound Med* 6: 475.

Chervenak FA, Issacson G, Mahoney MJ et al (1985) Diagnosis and management of fetal teratomas. *Obstet Gynecol* 66: 666–671.

Comstock CH & Kirk JS (1991) Arteriovenous malformations. Locations and evaluation in the fetal brain. *J Ultrasound Med* 10: 361–365.

Estroff JA, Parad RB, Barnes PD et al (1995) Posterior fossa arachnoid cyst: an in utero mimicker of Dandy–Walker malformation. *J Ultrasound Med* 14: 787–790.

Haimovici JA, Doubilet PM, Benson CB, Frates MC (1997) Clinical significance of isolated enlargement of cisterna magna (10 mm) or prenatal sonography. *J Ultra Med* 16: 731–734.

Hertzberg BS, Kliewer MA, Freed KS et al (1997) Third ventricle: size and appearance in normal fetuses through gestation. *Radiology* 203: 641–644.

Hertzberg BS, Kliewer MA & Provenzale JM (1997) Cyst of velum interpositum: antenatal ultrasonographic features and differential diagnosis. *J Ultra Med* 16: 767–770.

Keogan MT, DeAtinke AB & Hertzberg BS (1994) Cerebellar vermis defects: antenatal sonographic appearance and clinical significance. *J Ultra Med* 13: 607.

Komarniske CA, Cyr DR, Mack LA et al (1990) Prenatal diagnosis of schizencephaly. *J Ultrasound Med* 9: 305.

Meizner I & Elchalal U (1996) Prenatal sonographic diagnosis of anterior fossa porencephaly. *JCU* 24: 96–99.

Ostlers SJ, Irving JC & Liford RJ (1990) Fetal choroid plexus cysts. A report of 100 cases. *Radiology* 175: 753.

Patel MD, Goldstein RB, Tung S & Filly RA (1995) Fetal cerebral ventricular atrium: difference in size according to sex. *Radiology* 194: 713–715.

Pattern RM, Mark LA & Finberg HJ (1991) Unilateral hydrocephalus. Prenatal sonographic diagnosis. *AJR* 156: 359–363.

Russell SA (2000) Cranial abnormalities. In: *Textbook of fetal abnormalities*. Twining P, McHugo JM & Pilling DW (eds). Churchill Livingstone, London, pp 89–138

Shipp TD, Chu GC & Benacerraf B (2000) Prenatal diagnosis of Oral-Facial-Digital syndrome, Type I. *J Ultra Med* 19: 491–494.

Twining P, Zuccolla J, Clewes J & Swallow J (1991) Fetal choroid plexus cysts: a prospective study and review of the literature. *Br J Radiol* 64: 98–102.

Van Zalen-Sprock R, van Vug JMG, van der Harten HJ et al (1995) First trimester diagnosis of cyclopia and holoprosencephaly. *J Ultrasound Med* 14: 631–633.

Fetal Intracranial Bright Reflectors and Echogenic Masses

Physiologic

Choroid plexus

At around 17 weeks gestation the choroid plexus may fill most of the lateral ventricle. The fetal brain at this gestation is relatively sonolucent.

Leptomeninges

The leptomeninges (pia mater) outline the outer surface of the high brain and are seen as highly reflectile. Surrounding the leptomeninges is CSF in the subarachnoid space. The echogenicity of this space depends upon the relative amounts of CSF/leptomeninges. The smaller cisterns may appear highly echogenic, while the larger cistern may have an echolucent appearance. Seen with particular clarity if an ossification abnormality of the skull vault occurs, e.g. osteogenesis imperfecta.

Specular reflection

This is an artifact, which occurs when the ultrasound beam strikes the walls of the ventricles in a perpendicular/near perpendicular manner. The result is highly reflectile echoes emanating from the ventricular walls.

Reflections of unknown cause

Deep within the brain tissue, mostly in the region of the white matter, occasional high-amplitude echoes are noted. The way in which these are produced is unknown, but blood vessels, particularly penetrating veins, have been implicated.

Echogenic sulci

Sulci may appear echogenic in one plane but a change in the scanning plane by about 90° reveals normal sulci.

Reverberation artifact	A reverberation artifact in the near side of the fetal cranium is fairly common. This not only produces a pseudomass within the near side of the cranium but also prevents resolution of the proximal structures within the brain.
Pachymeninges	The falx and tentorium are components of the dura (pachymeninges), which also appear echogenic, making useful landmarks.
Cerebellar vermis	The cerebellar vermis lying in the posterior fossa below the tentorium may cause high-amplitude echoes. The fovea becomes visible as maturation occurs.

Pathologic

Cerebroventricular hemorrhage	When recent, hemorrhage within the brain parenchyma or ventricles may appear as an echogenic mass. Blood in the ventricular system may show a fluid–fluid level or echogenic clot. Follow-up sonography may show evolution of the hemorrhage progressing to liquefaction. Antenatal cerebellar hemorrhage has also been described presenting as a hyperechoic or hypoechoic cerebellar mass or cerebellar hemispheres of unequal size and echogenicity with the vermis not identified in one case. Ventriculomegaly is also associated. The cause is rarely identified but preeclampsia, thrombocytopenia, pancreatitis, maternal seizures and blood clotting abnormalities have been implicated.

Intracranial tumors – teratoma	Primary brain tumors are rare with an overall poor prognosis. Most are teratomas accounting for 50% of all brain tumors in the neonate. Teratomatous lesions tend to have mixed solid and cystic areas and they usually have a great degree of disorganization. Calcification is common. Most primary fetal brain tumors are supratentorial with variable echogenicity, have a mass effect, eccentric in location and may cause hydrocephalus. Without a biopsy it is usually not possible to offer a tissue diagnosis. Intracranial hemorrhage may mimic intracranial tumors but their changing US appearance from echogenic to hypoechoic/cystic on serial scans and lack of growth suggest a hemorrhage.
Choroid plexus papilloma	These are small benign tumors which arise from the normal choroid plexus. They are echogenic masses and can be differentiated from blood clot on serial scanning when the appearances remain constant.
Periventricular leukomalacia	This is caused by ischemia which may be hemorrhagic or non-hemorrhagic. The lesions affect the periventricular region, corona radiata and occipital area. The lesions change with time, becoming cystic.
Calcification	Calcification within the brain of a fetus may be related to transplacental infection. Echogenicity is seen in the periventricular region. Calcification may be seen in tuberose sclerosis.
Arteriorvenous malformation	AVMs usually present a cystic appearance but small compact AVMs may be highly reflectile because of the multiple interfaces. Diagnosis may be achieved by color Doppler sonography.

Sturge–Weber syndrome

SWS or trigeminal angiomatosis is associated with vascular malformations of the cerebral cortex and face. Even before the angiomatous malformation overlying the cortex calcifies, the leptomeninges show increased echogenicity.

Lipomas

Most intracranial lipomas occur near the midline: the majority are sited in the corpus callosum, in or below the third ventricle in the cerebellum, the cerebellopontine angle, over the quadrigeminal plate or in the sylvian fissure. Sonographically they appear as hyperechoic, smoothly marginated masses. They do not normally cause acoustic shadowing.

Glioblastoma

These tumours may present as focal, homogeneous hyperechoic or hypoechoic intracerebral masses associated with a mass effect and hydrocephalus.

Craniopharyngioma

A craniopharyngioma has been detected antenatally; this tumor replaced all the normal brain but had a different echo pattern. The mass was calcified and lobulated, and was surrounded by fluid.

Dermoid or epidermoid cyst

Appear as well marginated echogenic mass.

Cerebral neuroblastoma

This has been detected antenatally and diagnosed by a fetal brain biopsy. The lesion presented as a solid heterogeneous mass containing calcification, occupying the right cerebral hemisphere with a midline shift to the left. A large subdural fluid collection was also detected.

Intracranial Tumors that have been Detected Antenatally

- Teratomas – most common – cystic/solid component
- Meningeal sarcoma
- Craniopharyngioma
- Lipoma of the corpus callosum
- Oligodendroglioma
- Gangliocytoma

These tumours cannot be distinguished from each other until biopsy.

Further Reading

Belfar HL, Kuller JA, Hill LM et al (1991) Evolving fetal hydranencephaly mimicking intracranial neoplasm. *J Ultrasound Med* 10: 231.

Chung SN, Rosemond RL & Graham D (1998) Prenatal diagnosis of a fetal intracranial tumour. *J Ultrasound Med* 17: 521–523.

Guibaud L, Champion F, Buenerd A et al (1997) Fetal intraventricular glioblastoma: ultrasonographic, magnetic resonance imaging and pathologic findings. *J Ultrasound Med* 16: 285–288.

Mulligan G & Meier P (1989) Lipoma and agenesis of the corpus callosum with associated choroid plexus lipomas. *J Ultrasound Med* 8: 583.

Ranzini AG, Shen-Schwarz S & Guzman ER (1998) Prenatal sonographic appearance of hemorrhagic cerebellar infarction. *J Ultrasound Med* 17: 725–727.

Slovis TL, Shkoinic A & Hallor JD (1989) Focal areas of increased echogenicity within the brain biopsy. *J Ultrasound Med* 5: 303–306.

Winter TC, Laing FC, Mack LA & Born DE (1992) Prenatal sonographic diagnosis of a pontine lipoma. *J Ultrasound Med* 11: 559–561.

Differential Diagnosis of the 'Lemon Sign' in the Fetal Skull

Meningomyelocele

The 'lemon sign' describes scalloping of the fetal frontal bones in axial view at the level of BPD. When seen with meningomyelocele it is usually associated with Arnold–Chiari type II or III malformation with an abnormal cerebellar position. The positive predictive value of the 'lemon' sign in a low-risk population is 6%.

Normal fetus

The incidence quoted varies from 0.66 to 1.3%. No associated intracranial abnormality is apparent, i.e. normal-sized ventricle and normal cerebellum. The spine is normal.

Encephalocele

This is a part of the spectrum of neural tube defects and is often associated with type II or III Arnold–Chiari malformation. The majority of these are occipital in location. Rarely they may occur in the frontal region where themselves may mimic a 'lemon sign.'

Further Reading

Ball RH, Filly RA, Goldstein RB & Callen PW (1993) The lemon sign: not a specific indicator of meningomyelocele. *J Ultrasound Med* 3: 131–134.

van den Hof MC, Nicolaides KH, Campbell J et al (1990) Evaluation of the lemon and banana signs in one hundred and thirty fetuses with open spina bifida. *Am J Obstet Gynecol* 162: 322.

Dandy–Walker Malformation

'Classic'
Triad of cystic dilatation of the fourth ventricle, communicating with the posterior fossa cyst; complete or partial agenesis of the cerebellar vermis; enlarged posterior fossa with displacement of the tentorium, torcular and lateral sinus.

Dandy–Walker variant
Cerebellar dysgenesis with varying degrees of hypoplasia of the cerebellar vermis with normal-sized posterior fossa. Ventricular dilatation may occur. The cerebellar hemispheres may be hypoplastic.

Mega-cisterna magna
An enlarged cisterna magna with a normal cerebellar vermis and fourth ventricle. The cerebellum may be hypoplastic.

Associated anomalies
Associated anomalies occur in 70% of cases of Dandy–Walker malformation. These include: corpus callosum dysgenesis, subependymal neuronal heterotopia, polymicrogyria, agyria, schizencephaly, lipoma of corpus callosum, encephalocele, lumbosacral meningocele, vermian hypoplasia and posterior fossa dermoid cyst. Chromosomal abnormalities are also associated.

Further Reading

Altman NR, Naidch TP & Braffman BH (1992) Posterior fossa malformations. *AJNR* 13: 691–724.

Barkovich AJ, Kyos BD, Norman D & Edwards MS (1989) Revised classification of posterior fossa cysts and cyst like malformations based on the result of multiplane MR imaging. *AJNR* 10: 977–988.

Estroff JA, Scorf MR & Benacerraf BR (1992) Dandy–Walker variant: prenatal sonographic features and clinical outcome. *Radiology* 183: 755–758.

4

Fetal Face and Neck

Frontal bossing of forehead

Frontal bossing of the forehead is associated with many syndromes including skeletal dysplasias (achondroplasia, achondrogenesis, and thanatophoric dysplasia), Crouzon, Hurler, Pfeiffer, Robinson, Russell syndromes and craniofrontonasal dysplasia. Frontal bossing is best appreciated in the sagittal plane, where the relationship of the forehead and midface is seen to advantage.

Premaxillary protrusion

The abnormality may occur with complete cleft lip and palate and is usually seen with other types of facial clefting. Sonographically the PMP may be more obvious than the underlying cleft and may be an important clue to diagnosis.

Probosces in holoprosencephaly

A proboscis may be sited above a single median orbit (cyclopia) or as a fleshy primitive nose with a single nostril but normally sited. The fetus may have two orbits, have hypotelorism with associated probosces and an absent nose (cebocephaly). Midline facial clefting has also been recorded. Significant association with chromosome abnormality.

Cyclopia	Cyclopia is seen in association with holoprosencephaly in 10–20% of fetuses. In most cases the ocular fusion is incomplete and the fused eyes can be identified within one orbit. The nose is placed above the solitary midline orbit in the form of probosces. The mouth may be small or absent and the ears low-set.
Ethmocephaly	This an uncommon anomaly associated with holoprosencephaly and comprises of severe hypotelorism and a proboscis at the level of the orbits.
Teratoma	Teratomas (other than epignathus) may occur on the facial surface and in common with other teratomas present as a complex mass on sonography with some cystic elements. They may calcify. Nasopharyngeal teratoma may present with PH raised MSAFP and may prevent fusion of palatal processes resulting in clefting. Teratomas may present with high output failure secondary to AV shunting. Color Doppler may demonstrate arterial signal within the tumor.
Anterior encephalocele/ meningocele	These represent either herniation of meninges through a calvarial defect (cranial meningocele) or the herniation of brain and meninges (true encephalocele). The majority occur in the frontal midline. Absence of brain tissue within a cranial meningocele is an important favorable prognostic sign.
Enlarged protruding tongue	This may be associated with a tumor such as a teratoma or may occur as part of an organomegaly syndrome (Beckwith–Wiedemann). Beckwith–Wiedemann syndrome is associated with omphalocele, macroglossia gigantism, pancreatic hyperplasia and PH. There is an increased incidence of Wilms' tumors and hepatoblastomas.

Hemangioma	Hemangiomas can occur anywhere in the body. They may present as mixed or solid masses. Actual flow or pulsations help to identify their origin. Duplex Doppler may be diagnostic.
Epignathus	This is a benign teratomatous tumor arising from the sphenoid, nose, pharynx, tongue or jaw. The sonographic appearances are those of a lobular complex mass, primarily solid but with some cystic components. They may contain calcification.
Exophthalmos	This has been reported in association with Crouzon's syndrome (craniofacial dysostosis); other features of the syndrome include a deformed skull, mandibular prognathism, small maxilla, ocular hypertelorism and hydrocephalus.
Dacryocystocele	A lacrimal duct cyst which can be identified as a small hypoechoic mass inferomedial to the orbit. They do not have a mass effect on the orbit and most resolve spontaneously after birth.
Retinoblastoma	Uncommon tumor of childhood arising in the retina, which can occur at any age but 80% occur before the age of 5 years, it is hereditary in 40%, unilateral in 70% or bilateral in 30%. Hereditary retinoblastoma may be unilateral or bilateral, most unilateral tumors are not hereditary but all bilateral tumors are hereditary. US appearances in utero are those of a solid orbital mass deforming the face and brain and may cause hydrocephalus when the tumor spreads into the brain. The differential diagnosis is from a teratoma.

Oral granular cell myoblastoma | Congenital epulis usually situated in the alveolar ridge, predominantly in the maxilla varies in size from a few mm to cm, which may be broad-based or pedunculated. Benign tumor of unknown histologic origin. Intrabuccal tumor is rare. US features have been reported as showing parted lips, no clefting with a solid mass protruding attached to the mandible. Doppler US shows arterial flow arising from the base of attachment. Obstruction of the mouth may cause PH.

Harlequin ichthyosis | Autosomal recessive skin disorder associated with skin thickening and fissuring. The mouth is held fixed and is 'O'-shaped, cystic masses anterior to the orbits are typically seen because of pronounced ectropion. The lips also appear thickened and everted (eclabium).

Causes of Micrognathia

Mild forms of isolated micrognathia are often overlooked during routine antenatal US scanning. More severe forms of the anomaly are often associated with over 50 syndromes and chromosomal anomalies. The more common causes include:

- Chromosomal anomalies – Trisomies 18, 13, 9 and Triploidy 22 Trisomy/tetrasomy
- Musculoskeletal disease:

    Arthrogryposis
    Achondrogenesis
    Camptomelic dysplasia
    Diastrophic dysplasia
    Short rib polydactyly syndrome
    Atelosteogenesis
    Robinow syndrome

- Non-chromosomal syndromes

    Pierre–Robin syndrome
    Treacher–Collins syndrome
    Goldenhar syndrome (hemifacial microsomia)
    Pena–Shokeir syndrome
    Beckwith–Wiedemann syndrome
    Escobar syndrome
    Seckel syndrome
    DiGeorge syndrome
    Hydrolethalus syndrome
    Miller syndrome
    Mohr syndrome
    Cerebro-costo-mandibular syndrome
    Dubowitz syndrome
    Hallermann–Streiff syndrome
    Mobius syndrome
    Larsen syndrome
    Potter sequence
    Otocephaly*
    Oral-facial-digital syndrome type I

* May cause agnathia, antenatal differentiation between agnathia and micrognathia may be difficult.

Further Reading

Bromley B & Benacerraf BR (1994) Fetal micrognathia: associated anomalies and outcome. *J Ultra Med* 13: 529–533.

Jones KL (1997) *Smith's recognisable patterns of human malformations*. London: WB Saunders.

Rahmani R, Dixon M, Chityat D et al (1998) Otocephaly: prenatal diagnosis. *J Ultra Med* 17: 595–598.

Satoh S, Takashima T, Takeuchi H et al (1995) Antenatal sonographic detection of proximal esophageal segment: specific evidence of congenital esophageal atresia. *JCU* 23: 419–423.

Turners G & Twinning P (1993) The facial profile in the diagnosis of fetal abnormalities. *Clin Radiol* 47: 389–395.

Vijayarghavan SB (1996) Antenatal diagnosis of esophageal atresia with transesophageal fistula. *J Ultra Med* 15: 417–419.

Facial Clefting

Cleft lip with and without cleft palate (CL-P) is the most common congenital anomaly involving the face – 1 in 1000 live births with a marked racial variability. The highest frequency is amongst the American Indians – 3.6 per 1000, 1.5–2.0 per 1000 in Asians and 0.5% amongst Blacks. Approximately 80% of infants with cleft lip also have a cleft palate. CL-P etiologically distinct from cleft palate alone. Siblings of patients with CL-P have an increased frequency of CL-P but not cleft palate alone, whereas siblings of patients with a cleft palate alone have an increased frequency of cleft palate but not CL-P.

Ultrasound classification of facial clefts

- Type 1: cleft lip without cleft palate – associated with other anomalies in 20% but there is no relationship with chromosomal anomaly.
- Type 2: unilateral cleft lip and palate – associated with other anomalies in 47% and chromosomal anomaly in 20% of patients.
- Type 3: bilateral cleft lip and palate – other anomalies in 55% and chromosomal anomalies in 30%.
- Type 4: midline cleft lip and palate is associated with other anomalies in all and chromosomal anomalies in 52%.
- Type 5: cleft associated with ABS or limb-body-wall complex, all patients have associated non-chromosomal anomalies.

Cleft Lip/Palate: Associated Lesions

Chromosomal anomalies

- Trisomy 18
- Trisomy 13
- Trisomy 15 partial
- Turner's syndrome 45X
- Mosaic trisomy 22

Fetal milieu and life line

- IUGR
- Hydrops
- Single umbilical artery
- Amniotic bands

CNS and face

- Alobar holoprosencephaly
- ACC
- Exencephaly
- Occipital encephalocele
- Dandy–Walker malformation
- Unilateral anophthalmia
- Micrognathia
- Low-set ears
- Frontonasal dysplasia (medial cleft syndrome)

Abdomen and the GIT

- Absent stomach
- Omphalocele

Cardiac

- Cardiac defects
- Pericardial effusion
- Ectopia cardia

Musculoskeletal

- Spinal defects
- Scoliosis
- Polydactyly
- Clenched hands
- Club feet
- Skeletal dysplasia
- Limb-body-wall complex

Genitourinary

- Hydronephrosis

Further Reading

Babcook CJ, McGahan JP & Chong BW (1996) Evaluation of fetal midface anatomy to facial clefts: use of US. *Radiology* 201: 113–118.

Bowerman RA (1993) Ultrasound of the fetal face. *Ultrasound Q* 11: 211–258.

Devonald KJ, Ellwood DA, Griffiths KA et al (1995) Volume imaging: three-dimensional appreciation of the fetal head and face. *J Ultrasound Med* 14: 919–925.

Mahoney BS & Hegg F (1991) The fetal face. In: Nyberg DA, Mahoney BS & Pretorius DH (eds) *Diagnostic Ultrasound of Fetal Anomalies,* pp 203–261. Chicago: Mosby-Year Book.

Meizner I, Shalev J, Mashiah R et al (2000) Prenatal ultrasonographic diagnosis of congenital oral granular cell myoblastoma. *J Ultra Med* 19: 337–339.

Mernagh JR, Mohide PT, Lappalainen RE & Fedoryshin JG (1999) Ultrasound assessment of fetal head and neck. *Radiographics* 19: S229–S241.

Monni G, Ibba RM, Olla G et al (1995) Color Doppler ultrasound and prenatal diagnosis of cleft palate. *JCU* 23: 189–191.

Nyberg DA, Mahoney BS & Kramer D (1992) Paranasal echogenic mass. Sonographic sign of bilateral complete cleft lip and palate before 20 menstrual weeks. *Radiology* 184: 757–759.

Nyberg DA, Sickler K, Hegge FN et al (1995) Fetal cleft lip with and without cleft palate: US classification and correlation with outcome. *Radiology* 195: 677–684.

Paladini D, Morra T, Guida F et al (1998) Prenatal diagnosis and perinatal management of lingual lymphangioma. *Ultra Obstet Gynecol* 11: 141.

Salim A, Wiknjosastro GH, Danukusumo D et al (1998) Fetal retinoblastoma. *J Ultra Med* 17: 717–720.

Shipp TD, Bromley B & Benacerraf BR (1995) The ultrasonographic appearance and outcome for fetuses with masses distorting the fetal face. *J Ultrasound Med* 14: 673–678.

Twinning P (2000) Abnormalities of the face and neck. In: *Textbook of fetal abnormalities,* Twinning P, McHugo M & Pilling DW (eds), pp 345–389. Churchill Livingstone, London.

Walsh G & Dubbins PA (1994) Antenatal sonographic diagnosis of a dacryocystocele. *JCU* 22: 457.

Whisson CC, Whyte A & Ziesing P (1994) Beckwith–Wiedemann syndrome: antenatal diagnosis. *Australas Radiol* 38(2): 130–131.

Nuchal Translucency

The presence of first-trimester nuchal translucency 3 mm or more is strongly associated with increased risk of an abnormal karyotype. If amniocentesis reveals a normal karyotype then a targeted US examination is indicated. The nuchal translucency may be septate or non-septated. Fetuses with a septated nuchal translucency have a higher risk of abnormal karyotype and other associated abnormalities. Nuchal translucency is a transient abnormality and to detect it a US needs to be undertaken at 10–14 weeks gestation.

Fetal abnormalities associated with increased nuchal translucency thickness

- Normal – 0.06%

- Chromosomal anomalies
  Trisomy 21 – 45–80%
  Turner's syndrome – 45XO
  Trisomy 18
  Noonan's syndrome
  Syndrome XXX, XXXX, XXXXY, XYY
  Syndrome 18p & 13q

- Non-chromosomal anomalies
  Cardiac defects
  Diaphragmatic hernia
  Exomphalos
  Body stalk anomaly

- Non-chromosomal syndromes
  Escobar syndrome (multiple pterygium syndrome)
  Skeletal dysplasias
  Klippel–Feil syndrome
  Zellweger syndrome
  Robert's syndrome
  Cumming's syndrome
  Joubert syndrome
  Meckel's syndrome
  Fryns syndrome
  Smith–Lemli–Opitz syndrome
  Hydrolethalus syndrome
  Spinal muscular atrophy
  Myotonic dystrophy
  Parovirus infection

Further Reading

Smulian JC, Egan JFX & Rodis JF (1998) Fetal hydrops in the first trimester associated with maternal parvovirus infection. *JCU* 26: 314–316.

van Vugt JMB, van Zalen-Sprock RM & Kostemse PJ (1996) First-trimester nuchal translucency: A risk analysis on fetal chromosomal abnormality. *Radiology* 200: 537–540.

Causes of Congenital Cataracts

- TORCH infections 36%

- Idiopathic 32%

- Enzyme defects 23%
  Galactosemia
  Galactokinase deficiency
  G6PD deficiency
  Homocystinuria

- Familial syndrome 9%
  Hallerman–Streiff
  Lowe's
  Alport's
  Conradi–Hünermann
  Smith-Lemli-Opitz

NB Congenital cataracts are seen in utero as (1) densely echogenic lenses, (2) as a double ring appearance where the outer ring represents the border of the lens and the inner ring the cataract, or (3) a central echogenic focus within the lens. Detection is usually achieved in the second trimester. The demonstration of clear lenses on sonography does not exclude the presence of congenital cataracts.

Further Reading

Gaary EA, Rawnsley E, Martin-Padilla JM et al (1993) In utero detection of fetal cataracts. *J Ultrasound Med* 4: 234–236.
Monteagudo A, Timor-Tritch IE, Friedman AH & Santos R (1996) Autosomal dominant cataracts of the fetus: early detection by transvaginal ultrasound. *Ultrasound Obstetrics Gynecol* 8: 104-108.

Craniostenosis Syndromes

Craniostenosis is characterized by premature fusion of cranial sutures and may occur as an isolated anomaly or as a part of more complex syndromes. The suture fusion may be symmetrical or less commonly asymmetrical. The skull shape depends upon the sutures involved in the process of premature fusion – elongated (dolicocephalic) skull with premature fusion of sagittal suture, rounded (brachycephalic), a pointed vertex (turrincephaly or acrocephaly) with coronal suture premature fusion and a clover-leaf skull when all the skull sutures fuse prematurely. Premature skull suture fusion is often associated with changes of raised intracranial pressure and or hydronephrosis.

Apert syndrome
: Is an autosomal dominant condition but most cases occur sporadically as a result of mutation. Craniostenosis is a prominent feature associated with turrincephaly prominent protruding eyes (proptosis), cleft palate, vertebral fusion, hydronephrosis, CHD (10%), brachydactyly and postaxial polydactyly of and syndactyly of the toes. Nearly half the children are mentally deficient.

Carpenter familial syndrome
: Autosomal recessive with intra-familial variability. The syndrome is characterized by acrocephaly, mid-face hypoplasia, flat facial profile – depressed nasal bridge, post-axial polydactyly in hands and pre-axial polydactyly in feet. Other reported abnormalities include CHD, clindactyly, camptodactyly, and umbilical hernia. Approximately 75% are mentally retarded.

Crouzon syndrome
: Autosomal dominant, but sporadic in about a quarter of the cases. Characterized by brachycephaly or oxycephaly and less commonly scaphocephaly and trigoncephaly, proptosis, hypertelorism, frontal bossing, mandibular prognathism, beaked nose and rarely cleft palate. Children usually have normal intelligence.

Pfeiffer syndrome	Autosomal dominant, characterized by skull and facial anomalies – acrocephaly; brachycephaly, clover-leaf skull, proptosis, hypertelorism, flattened nose, broad and duplicated big toes, broad thumbs with ulnar deviation and brachydactyly. Clover-leaf skull usually has a poor prognosis. There is mental deficiency in a minority of children.
Saethre–Chotzen syndrome	Autosomal dominant with a marked penetrance and variable expressivity, characterized by brachycephaly and/or acrocephaly, mid-face hypoplasia, hypertelorism, beaked nose, low-set ears, cleft palate, brachydactyly, partial or soft syndactyly and rarely CHD and renal anomalies. The majority of children have normal intelligence.
Craniofrontonasal dysplasia	Rare X-linked dominant disorder, with lethality in males characterized by brachycephaly, plagiocephaly, acrocephaly, dolichocephaly, frontal bossing, mid-face hypoplasia, cleft lip/palate and hypertelorism. The intelligence is usually normal.

Fetal Anophthalmia

Trisomy 13

The most important sonographic findings are in the head, face, heart and hands and include holoprosencephaly, ACC, SWS, hydrocephalus, anophthalmia, low-set ears, cleft lip/palate, VSD, ASD, PDA, pulmonary stenosis, mitral/aortic atresia, polydactyly, omphalocele and renal cystic dysplasia.

Goltz's syndrome

The syndrome is inherited in an X-linked dominant manner and may be associated with microphthalmia, unilateral anophthalmia, single umbilical artery, syndactyly, adactyly, polydactyly, microcephaly, foot deformities and renal anomalies.

Fraser's syndrome

(Cryptophthalmos-syndactyly syndrome) The syndrome is associated with various ocular abnormalities (absence of lens, abnormal size, absence of orbits), microcephaly, syndactyly, renal dysplasia and renal agenesis.

Goldenhar's syndrome

This is usually a sporadic condition, familial cases are rare. Sonographic features include anophthalmia, low-set ears, vertebral anomalies, intracranial anomalies, intracranial lipomas/dermoid, encephalocele, hydrocephalus, pulmonary agenesis, cleft palate and absence of the portal vein.

Lenz's microphthalmos syndrome

This is an X-linked recessive condition. Anophthalmia/microphthalmia, deformed ears, microcephaly, cleft lip/palate, webbed neck, renal anomalies, CHD, clindactyly, camptodactyly and syndactyly.

Waardenburg's anophthalmia syndrome

This syndrome is inherited in an autosomal recessive manner. It has not been reported antenatally. Expected features: anophthalmia/microphthalmos, syndactyly, camptodactyly and clubfeet.

Branchio-oculo-facial syndrome

Characterized by IUGR (50%) post-natal growth deficiency, ocular defects, lacrimal duct obstruction, microphthalmia or anophthalmia, abnormal lip – pseudo-cleft and various degrees of cleft micrognathia, low-set ears and premature aging. Antenatal diagnosis has been reported with bilateral cleft lip, clefting was unusual in that it did not extend into the nostrils but the nose was not distorted. The globes were not detected within the orbits (anophthalmia).

Fetal Microphthalmos

Phenylketonuria
Autosomal recessive condition associated with IUGR, MOPH; prenatal diagnoses can be achieved by amniocentesis and analysis of DNA isolated from amniotic cell culture.

Pena–Shokeir syndrome
(Cerebro-oculofacioskeletal syndrome) Sonographically may reveal PH, placentomegaly, hydrops fetalis, joint contractures/arthrogryposis, micrognathia, small narrow thoracic cavity, hypotelorism and MOPH.

Amniotic band syndrome
This is a non-inherited condition in which the amniotic bands cause slash defects. Anomalies of the face include asymmetrical clefts, anencephaly, microcephaly, encephalocele, microphthalmos and transient OH.

Fanconi anemia
Autosomal recessive; associated with limb anomalies, absent, hypoplastic or supernumerary thumbs, hypoplastic/absent radii, syndactyly, MOPH, microcephaly, renal aplasia, horse-shoe kidneys and hydronephrosis. Prenatal diagnosis may be confirmed by increase in chromosomal breakage in amniotic cells when exposed to diepoxybutane.

Fetal toxoplasmosis
Associated anomalies include microcephaly, MOPH, hydrops, IUGR, hydranencephaly, hydrocephalus secondary to aqueduct stenosis, porencephalic cyst and periventricular calcification. Hepatic and spleen calcification has been reported in the newborn.

Fetal rubella syndrome
Associated anomalies reported include craniostenosis, aqueduct stenosis, cysts of the subependymal germinal matrix, congenital cataract, MOPH, CHD, esophageal atresia, IUGR.

Fetal herpes simplex infection	Features include microcephaly, MOPH and IUGR. Cerebral, periventricular, liver and adrenal calcification have been reported in the neonate.
Fetal alcohol syndrome	This occurs in the fetuses of chronic alcoholic mothers. Associated features include MOPH, microcephaly, micrognathia, cleft lip/palate, CHD, hemangiomas, congenital tumors, diaphragmatic hernia and hydronephrosis.
Fetal isotretinoin syndrome	Isotretinoin is a teratogenic drug, reported to have caused holoprosencephaly, hydrocephalus, agenesis of the vermis, hypertelorism, MOPH, micrognathia, external ear anomalies and CHD.
Hydrolethalus syndrome	(Salonen–Herva–Norio syndrome) This is an autosomal recessive condition associated with MOPH, micrognathia deformed ears, cleft lip/palate postaxial polydactyly in hands, preaxial polydactyly in feet, CHD, omphalocele, PH, hydrocephalus, DWD, hypoplasia of tibias and bilateral pulmonary agenesis.
Roberts' syndrome	Inherited in an autosomal recessive manner, the syndrome is associated with IUGR, MOPH, hypertelorism, cataracts, frontal encephalocele, hydrocephalus, facial hemangioma, nuchal cystic hygroma, limb reduction anomaly, clindactyly, clubfeet, renal anomalies and CHD.
Meckel–Gruber syndrome	This is an autosomal recessive condition associated with occipital encephalocele, hydrocephalus, small BPD, MOPH, CHD, short limbs and cystic dysplasia, giving rise to large kidneys, absent bladder.
Treacher–Collins syndrome	This is an autosomal dominant condition associated with hypoagenesis/agenesis of the mandible, vertebral anomalies, MOPH, micrognathia, cleft palate, CHD and limb anomalies.

Median cleft face syndrome	(Fibronasal dysplasia) Most of these cases are autosomal recessive or dominant. The features associated include a median cleft of the nose and frontal bone, MOPH, hypertelorism, holoprosencephaly, hydrocephalus, choanal atresia, deformed anterior horns of the lateral ventricles, ACC, congenital cataracts, cleft lip/palate, meningocele, encephalocele, clindactyly, camptodactyly and CHD.
Warfarin embryopathy	Due to maternal warfarin ingestion. The low-molecular-weight warfarin crosses the placenta resulting in significant levels in the fetus. About 10% of infants born alive have embryopathy. The syndrome is associated with hypertelorism, MOPH, cataracts, nasal hypoplasia, depressed nasal bridge, large tongue, hydrocephalus, occipital meningocele, stippled vertebral bodies and femoral epiphyses, CHD, asplenia and limb reduction anomalies and IUGR. US features: combination of history of warfarin exposure and associated IUGR, ventriculomegaly, nasal hypoplasia, with depressed nasal bridge and stippling of vertebral and femoral epiphysis should suggest the diagnosis.
Thalidomide	Related to maternal ingestion of thalidomide early in pregnancy. The syndrome is unlikely to be seen in utero at the present time as the drug is no longer prescribed in pregnancy. The syndrome is associated with limb anomalies, MOPH, ear abnormalities, renal and intestinal malformation and CHD.
Goltz's syndrome	X-linked dominant condition associated with MOPH, unilateral anophthalmia, single umbilical artery, syndactyly, polydactyly, adactyly, microcephaly, renal anomalies and foot deformities.

Goldenhar's syndrome	This is a specific condition with rare familial cases. Features include anophthalmia, MOPH, ventricular anomalies, intracranial lipoma/ dermoid, anencephaly, hydronephrosis, pulmonary agenesis and cleft palate.
Holoprosencephaly	(1) *Alobar type*. This is the most severe, with a monoventricle, fused thalami, absence of falx and corpus callosum. The cerebral cortex is horseshoe-shaped and lies anteriorly. The dorsal cyst has no overlying brain cortex. (2) *Semilobar type*. There is a monoventricle with a rudimentary occipital horn, which communicates with a dorsal sac. The thalami are partially fused. (3) *Lobar type*. The lateral ventricles are fused anteriorly but separated into the occipital horns. The lateral horns are enlarged anteriorly and communicate in the midline.
Hallermann–Streiff syndrome	(Oculomandibulofacial syndrome) Associated features include MOPH, congenital cataracts, low-set ears, micrognathia, small pinched nose, microstomia, scaphocephaly or brachycephaly (BPD anomalies).
CHARGE syndrome	Autosomal dominant or recessive; associated with MOPH, atresia of choana, PH, CHD, CNS anomalies, ear anomalies, deafness, TOF and VATER association.
Cohen's syndrome	Probably autosomal recessive; association with MOPH, microcephaly, hypotelorism, micrognathia, prominent ears, syndactyly, thoracic scoliosis, IUGR.

Aplasia cutis congenita	(Adams–Oliver syndrome) Autosomal recessive, rarely autosomal dominant; features demonstrable on ultrasound include microphthalmia, meningocele, hydrocephalus, TOF, hemangiomas and hands/feet/digit anomalies. The skin and scalp lesions are usually not detectable on sonography.
Bardet–Biedl syndrome	Autosomal recessive; associated with polydactyly, syndactyly, clindactyly of the 5th finger, urogenital anomalies (hydronephrosis) and CHD.
Fetal varicella syndrome	Abnormalities reported include IUGR, microcephaly, MOPH, congenital cataract, hypoplasia of limbs, digits, mandible and ribs, equinovarus and calcaneovalgus, hydrocephalus, cerebral hypoplasia, spinal scoliosis, GIT and genitourinary anomalies. Basal ganglia calcification has been reported in the newborn.
Hypopituitarism	In the fetus and neonate this is likely to be related to familial condition (autosomal recessive or X-linked recessive) congenital absence of the pituitary gland or secondary to a craniopharyngioma. The fetal sonographic features are likely to present as MOPH, IUGR and postaxial polydactyly. An intracranial mass lesion such as craniopharyngioma may be seen. Congenital hypopituitarism has not yet been reported on antenatal sonography.
Incontinentia pigmentis	(Block–Sulzberger syndrome) This X-linked dominant condition is lethal in males. Associated features include a single umbilical artery, MOPH, microcephaly, hydrocephalus, porencephalic cyst, clubfeet, cataracts, syndactyly and vertebral anomalies.

Kenny–Caffey syndrome

(Tubular stenosis dysplasia) This is an X-linked condition; most features of the syndrome become evident postnatally, antenatal diagnosis is therefore likely to be difficult but with a positive family history features like IUGR, MOPH and macrocephaly may point to an affected fetus.

Lenz's microphthalmos syndrome

The features of this recessive X-linked condition include anophthalmos, MOPH, microcephaly, cleft lip/palate, webbed neck, deformed ears, renal anomalies, CHD and anomalies of finger and toes.

Neu–Laxova syndrome

This is an autosomal recessive condition associated with IUGR, hypoechoic skeleton, kyphosis, microcephaly, receding forehead, protuberant eyes, MOPH, absent digits, short hands, 'sickle-like' long bones, flexion deformaties, rockerbottom feet, syndactyly, micrognathia, deformed ears, PH or OH.

Oculodento-osseous dysplasia

This is an autosomal dominant condition with a variable expressivity associated with MOPH, clindactyly of the 5th finger, syndactyly and camptodactyly of the 4th and 5th fingers, cleft lip/palate, small orbits, hypotelorism, wide mandible and hypoplasia/absence of phalanges of toes and fingers.

Osteoporosis-pseudoglioma syndrome

This is an autosomal recessive condition associated with MOPH, cataracts, microcephaly, kyphoscoliosis, CHD (VSD).

Pallister–Hall syndrome

This syndrome is associated with MOPH, microcephaly, hypothalamic hamartoblastoma, renal agenesis and/or renal dysplasia, imperforate anus, postaxial polydactyly, CHD and IUGR. The syndrome has not yet been diagnosed antenatally.

Proteus syndrome	The characteristics of the syndrome are asymmetric focal overgrowth, macrocephaly, macrodactyly of the hands and feet, subcutaneous vascular tumor, warty pigmented nevi and lipoid visceral tumors. Prenatal ultrasonic findings include hypertrophy and subcutaneous cysts in an extremity, macrodactyly, MOPH, cataracts and intra-abdominal masses (lipomas and lymphangiomas.)
Pseudohypo–parathyroidism	This is normally an X-linked condition. Most clinical features develop in early childhood/adult life. MOPH is a congenital feature and may conceivably be detected antenatally.
Scapuloiliac dysostosis	Probably autosomal dominant; only four cases have been reported. Expected sonographic features will include MOPH, hypertelorism, low-set ears, micrognathia, cranium bifidum, clindactyly of fingers and simple partial syndactyly.
Cat's eye syndrome	Associated with partial tetrasomy for 22q11 in most cases. Facial anomalies include MOPH, ocular hypertelorism, low-set ears; anorectal abnormalities may occur including Hirschsprung's disease and/or atresia.

Fetal Hypotelorism

NB In hypotelorism the interorbital distance is reduced. Hypotelorism per se is very rare.

Holoprosencephaly — The most common cause of hypotelorism is holoprosencephaly, although both these conditions are comparatively rare. Anomalies of the orbits, nose, median upper lip and palate occur.

Trisomy 21 — Associated features include increased nuchal fold, duodenal atresia, omphalocele, cystic hygroma, CHD, hypoplasia of the middle phalanx of the 5th finger, increased space between the 1st and 2nd toes and hydrops fetalis.

Williams' syndrome — Inherited as autosomal dominant with variable expressivity, the features associated include CHD and several cardiovascular anomalies, micrognathia, hypotelorism, 5th finger clindactyly, camptodactyly, talipes equinovarus, kyphoscoliosis and pulmonary sequestration.

Phenylketonuria — Hypotelorism in the fetus may be related to fetal effects of maternal phenylketonuria.

Trisomy 13 — Holoprosencephaly may occur as a part of trisomy 13. The most important sonographic findings of this condition are in the face, head, heart and hands. The facial anomalies include a cleft lip/palate and low-set ears.

Meckel's syndrome — This autosomal recessive condition is associated with occipital encephalocele, hydrocephalus, short limbs, CHD and dysplastic kidneys.

DiGeorge's syndrome
: Autosomal dominant; associated with hypoplastic mandible, low-set ears, hyper/hypotelorism, cleft lip/palate, CHD, TOF, imperforate anus, hypocalcemic tetany and infections in the newborn.

Fetal hydantoin syndrome
: This syndrome is related to maternal ingestion of the anticonvulsant drug, hydantoin. Associated features include microcephaly, low-set ears, cleft lip/palate, limb anomalies, CHD, diaphragmatic hernia and cystic hygroma.

Craniosynostosis
: Associated features include dysplastic ears, hypotelorism/hypertelorism, cleft lip/palate, facial capillary hemangioma, craniosynostosis, radical aplasia, fibular aplasia, hand/foot and vertebral anomalies.

Microcephaly
: Microcephaly is associated with many syndromes and environmental factors resulting in insult to the developing brain, e.g. infection, drugs. Diagnosis may be difficult as microcephaly may not develop until late in pregnancy. Poor head growth leads to a decline in the head:abdomen ratios.

Oculodental dysplasia
: Inherited in an autosomal dominant manner with variable expressivity, associated features include syndactyly, camptodactyly, clindactyly, phalanx aplasia, dysplasia or hypoplasia, cleft lip/palate, microphthalmos, hypotelorism and a thin nose.

Trigonocephaly
: The condition is inherited as autosomal dominant; associated features include trigonocephaly, due to premature fusion of metopic sutures, hypotelorism, omphalocele, hemivertebrae and minor malformations of fingers and toes.

Chromosome 18p
syndrome

This syndrome is caused by deletion of the short arm of chromosome 18. Most features of this condition may be difficult to detect antenatally. The features include craniofacial dysmorphism, hypo/hypertelorism, small chin, big protruding ears, kyphoscoliosis and curved 5th finger. The characteristics are obvious after birth.

Chromosome 5p
syndrome

Associated features include IUGR, micrognathia, microcephaly, hypertelorism, low-set ears, CHD, scoliosis and small iliac wings.

Otocephaly

Severe first and second arch defects non-familial, rare often lethal syndrome, characterized by severe mandibular hypoplasia or agnathia, synotia (ventromedial displacement of external ears) and microstomia. US features are those of multiple anomalies of fetal face, agnathia, sloped forehead, low-set ears, hypotelorism and hypoplasia of the molar areas and PH.

Fetal Hypertelorism

Hypertelorism is defined clinically as increased distance between the pupils. It is detected sonographically by measuring the distance between orbits. Both intraocular and extraocular distance can be measured against the mean, it is easy to determine the degree of hypertelorism. Dysmorphic facial features can easily be observed. A multitude of syndromes are associated with hypertelorism, and most have in common cranial contour abnormalities, such as those caused by craniosynostosis. Most of these syndromes are also associated with limb and digit anomalies. Hypoplastic greater wings of the sphenoid and overgrowth of the lesser wings of the sphenoid are said to be responsible for the defect. Overgrowth of the nasofrontal process of the frontal encephalocele may space the orbits wide apart and prevent them from reaching their normal anatomical position.

Frontal bossing of skull

- Gorlin's syndrome (basal nevus syndrome)
- Craniofrontonasal dysplasia
- Craniometaphyseal dysplasia
- Otopalatodigital syndrome type 1
- Robinow's syndrome
- Sclerosteosis
- Warfarin syndrome

Brachycephaly (Apert type)

- Cleidocranial dysostosis
- Acrocephalosyndactyly
- Brachiogenitoskeletal syndrome

Dolichocephaly

- Noonan's syndrome (also macrocephaly)
- G syndrome
- Marden's syndrome (also cleft lip)

Broad/square forehead

- Treacher–Collins syndrome
- Camptomelic dysplasia
- Larsen's syndrome (also cleft palate and uvula)
- Chromosome 18p syndrome (broad nose, flat face)
- Coffin–Lowry syndrome
- Opitz–Kaveggia syndrome

Mass lesion forehead/mid upper face

- Cleft lip
- Median cleft face syndrome
- Meckel's syndrome
- Anterior encephalocele
- Roberts' syndrome
- DiGeorge's syndrome
- Bifid nose
- Glioma of nose
- Chromosome 4p –
- Nose and nasal septum defect
- Fetal hydantoin syndrome

Delayed cranial ossification

- Ehlers–Danlos syndrome (flat orbit)

Aarskog syndrome — X-linked large variability of expression and share several phenotypic manifestations with other genetic conditions such as Noonan's syndrome, craniofrontonasal dysplasia, Robinow and Opitz syndromes. The syndrome is manifest by a short stature, structural anomalies of face, distal extremities and external genitalia. The facial anomalies include hypertelorism, broad forehead, broad nasal bridge, short nose with everted nostrils, widow's peak hair anomaly, ocular and ear anomalies, webbed neck and cystic hygroma. Musculoskeletal abnormalities include short broad hands, polydactyly, interdigital webbing, hypoplasia of the middle phalanges, proximal interphalangeal laxity with concomitant flexion and restriction of movement of the distal interphalangeal joints, flat broad feet, bulbous toes and spinal defects.

Frontonasal dysplasia	Sporadic disorder: occasional familial autosomal dominant, poorly defined syndrome – midline facial defects, involving orbits, forehead and nose. The facial characteristics include hypertelorism, bifid nose, broad nasal bridge, midline deficit of frontal bone and extension of the frontal hairline to form widow's peak.
Jacobsen syndrome	Deletion of distal long arm of chromosome 11 (distal 11q monosomy). Moderately to severely retarded, trigoncephaly, prominent forehead, upturned nose, depressed nasal bridge and carp-like mouth. Associated with CHD – ASD/VSD coarctation of aorta, pyloric stenosis, genitourinary anomalies and short stature. Couples with one partner carrying a balanced translocation appear to have a high spontaneous miscarriage rate. There is an 11% risk of producing an offspring with an unbalanced chromosomal complement. Therefore genetic counselling and prenatal diagnosis should be offered to the couple. US: PH, trigoncephaly, hypertelorism, micrognathia and prominent anteverted nose.

Further Reading

Auerbach AD, Sagi M & Alder B (1985) Fanconi anemia. Prenatal diagnoses in 30 fetuses at risk. *Pediatrics* 76: 794–800.

Aughton DJ & Cassidy SB (1987) Hydrolethalus syndrome: report of an apparent mild case, literature review and differential diagnosis. *Am J Med Genet* 27: 935–942.

Blane CE, Holt JF & Vine K (1984) Scapuloiliac dysostosis. *Br J Radiol* 57: 526–528.

Bromley B, Miller WA, Mansour R & Benacerraf BR (1998) Prenatal findings of Branchio-Oculo-Facial syndrome. *J Ultra Med* 17: 475–477.

Bronshtein M, Zimmer E, Gersoni-Baruch R et al (1991) First and second trimester diagnosis of fetal ocular defects and associated anomalies: report of eight cases. *Obstet Gynecol* 77: 443.

Burkett G (1983) Perinatal infections. *J Fla Med Assoc* 70: 749.

Buyes ML (ed.) *Birth Defects Encyclopedia.* Cambridge: Blackwell Scientific.

Cardwall MS (1987) Pena-Shokeir syndrome: prenatal diagnoses by ultrasonography. *J Ultrasound Med* 6: 619–621.

Crane JP & Beaver HA (1986) Midtrimester sonographic diagnosis of mandibulo-facial dysostosis. *Am J Med Genet* 25: 231–255.

Culler FL & Jones KL (1984) Hypopituitarism in association with post-axial polydactyly. *J Pediatr* 104: 881–884.

Davenport SJH, Hefner MA & Mitchell JA (1986) The spectrum of clinical features in CHARGE syndrome. *Clin Genet* 29: 298–310.

Frattarelli JL, Boley TJ, Miller RA (1996) Prenatal diagnosis of frontonasal dysplasia (median cleft syndrome). *J Ultra Med* 15: 81–85.

Graham JM Jr, Stephens TD & Shepard TH (1983) Nuchal cystic hygroma in a fetus with presumed Roberts' syndrome. *Am J Med Genet* 15: 163 (letter).

Hall JG (1986) Invited editorial comment. Analysis of Pena-Shokeir phenotype. *Am J Med Genet* 25: 99–117.

Hall JG, Pallister PD, Claren SK et al (1981) Congenital hypothalamic hamarto-blastoma, hypopituitarism, imperforate anus and post-axial polydactyly. A new syndrome? Clinical, causal and pathologic considerations. *Am J Med Genet* 7: 47.

Kuster W, Lenz W, Kaariainen H et al (1989) Congenital scalp defects with distal limb anomalies (Adams–Oliver syndrome). Report of ten cases and review of the literature. *Am J Med Genet* 31: 99–115.

Lammar EJ, Chen DT, Hoar RM et al (1985) Retinoic acid embryopathy. *N Engl J Med* 313: 837–841.

Laron Z (1986) Pituitary insufficiency in cleft palate or lip. *Am J Med Genet* 24: 547 (letter).

Lon IT, Lott IT, Boccin M et al (1984) Fetal hydrocephalus and ear anomalies associated with maternal use of isotretinoin. *J Pediatr* 105: 597–600.

McArthur RG, Morgan K, Philips JA et al (1985) Pre-natal diagnoses of Pena-Shokeir syndrome type I. *Am J Genet* 21: 279.

Mahboubi S & Templeton JM (1984) Association of Hirschsprung's disease and im-perforate anus in a patient with 'cat-eye' syndrome. *Pediatr Radiol* 14: 441–442.

Muller LM, de-Long G, Mouton SC et al (1987) A case of the Neu–Laxova syndrome: prenatal ultrasonographic monitoring in the third trimester and the histo-pathological findings. *Am J Med Genet* 26: 421–429.

O'Brien JE & Feingold M (1985) Incontinentia pigmenti: a longitudinal study. *Am J Dis Child* 139: 711–712.

Rabinowicz IM (1981) New ophthalmic findings in fetal syndrome. *JAMA* 245: 108.

Rahmani R, Dixon M, Chityat D et al (1998) Otocephaly: prenatal diagnosis. *J Ultra Med* 17: 595-598.

Richard DS, Williams CA, Cruz AC et al (1991) Prenatal sonographic findings in a fetus with proteus syndrome. *J Ultrasound Med* 10: 47-50.

Romke C, Froster-Ishenius U & Heyne K (1987) Robert's syndrome and SC phocomelia. A single genetic entity. *Clin Genet* 31: 170-177.

Salnen R, Henva R & Norio R (1981) The hydrolethalus syndrome. Delineation of a 'new' lethal malformation syndrome based on 28 patients. *Clin Genet* 19: 321.

Scott CI, Louro JM, Laurenc KM et al (1981) Comments on the Neu-Laxova syndrome and CAD complex. *Am J Med Genet* 9: 165.

Strerissguth AP, Clarren SK & Jones KL (1985) Natural history of the fetal alcohol syndrome: a 10 year follow-up of eleven patients. *Lancet* ii: 85.

Tayabi H & Lachman RS (1996) *Radiology of Syndromes, Metabolic Disorders and Skeletal Dysplasias*, 4th edn. Chicago: Year Book Medical.

Tongsong T, Wanapirak C & Piyamongkol W (1999) Prenatal ultrasonographic findings consistent with fetal warfarin syndrome. *J Ultra Med* 18: 577-580.

Wax JR, Smith JF, Floyd RC, Eggleston MK (1995) Prenatal ultrasonographic findings associated with Jacobsen syndrome. *J Ultra Med* 14: 256-258.

Yagopsky P, Reoveni H, Karplus M et al (1986) Aplasia cutis congenita in one of monozygotic twins. *Pediatr Dermatol* 8: 403-405.

Young ID & Moore JR (1987) Intrafamilial variation in Cohen syndrome. *J Med Genet* 24: 488-492.

Fetal Neck Masses

Cystic hygroma

Cystic hygromas are multiseptate cystic masses, often bilateral, located posterolaterally along the neck. The majority (75%) are associated with abnormal karyotypes, therefore a karyotyping procedure is appropriate. CH is associated with trisomies 21, 18 and 13 and several syndromes including Turner's, Noonan's, Roberts', Cumming's, Lowchock's, Aarskog syndrome and lethal multiple pterygium. It has also been reported with achondrogenesis type II and teratogens such as alcohol, aminopterin and trimethadone. PH and hydrops are frequently associated. They tend to regress as pregnancy advances. In a karyotypically normal fetus with no associated US abnormalities the outcome is usually good.

Pseudomembrane

Described by Hertzberg et al, it is felt to be secondary specular reflection from the developing skin on the back of the neck in early pregnancy. This 'artifact' is difficult to differentiate from small CH. However, a pseudomembrane is usually seen in fetuses in a 'neck up' position, and is seldom multiseptate. It is thought that at least some of the CH detected at 9-15 weeks and which showed spontaneous resolution may be related to a 'pseudomembrane.'

Nuchal thickening

Nuchal skin thickening is measured on an axial plane which includes the cisterna magna and the cavum septum pellucidum. The nuchal skin is regarded as abnormally thick if the distance between the calvarium and the dorsal skin boundary is 6 mm or greater in the second trimester, and indicates the need for karyotyping. The anomaly accompanies various chromosomal aberrations, particularly trisomy 21, Escobar's and Zellweger's syndromes and Klippel-Feil sequence.

Goiter

This may present as a solid bilobed mass with some echolucent areas. Its location will suggest its origin. Typical appearances and location will not cause confusion with teratomas. However, thyroid teratoma diagnosed as goiter has been described. Fetal goiter may decrease in size with maternal treatment. Causes of fetal goiter include maternal ingestion of iodides, maternal ingestion of anti-thyroid drugs, endemic iodine deficiency and autosomal recessive enzyme deficiency.

Hemangioma

Hemangiomas can occasionally appear in the neck region. They usually have a mixed or solid appearance. Actual pulsations or flow helps to identify their origin. Duplex Doppler is a useful adjunct.

Branchial cleft cyst

This represents an anterolateral neck mass, usually cystic and unilocular. There are usually no associated anomalies.

Teratoma

This neck mass may be cystic, mixed or solid and may show continuous growth in utero. The masses are usually benign and present as a lobular complex appearance. Calcification is frequent. Associated anomalies include hemangiomas, branchial cysts and PH.

Neuroblastoma	Neuroblastoma metastases to the subcutaneous tissues of the neck have been detected antenatally; these metastases should not be confused with a goiter because of the asymmetric placement.
Encephalocele	This is usually an occipital mass but may be low enough to enter the differential diagnosis of a neck mass. Demonstration of a bony defect is necessary to make a diagnosis. Associated ventricular dilatation may be evident.
Thyroglossal cyst	Thyroglossal cyst is usually a unilocular mass which presents in the midline and, unlike a teratoma, has no solid elements.
Sarcoma	Undifferentiated sarcoma has been detected antenatally. It presents as a solid unilateral neck mass with PH.
Klippel–Trenaunay–Weber syndrome	A large multiloculated mass in the anterior neck has been reported in utero, associated with subcutaneous cystic lesion in an extremity.
Cervical meningocele	This is associated with a spinal arch abnormality.
Nuchal translucency	Measured from the cervical vertebrae to the skin surface, >3 mm at 10–16 weeks has an increased incidence of aneuploidy. Karyotyping should be considered.
Non-fusion of the amnion	This should not be confused with nuchal translucency.
Congenital esophageal atresia	Congenital esophageal atresia may give rise to an anechoic area in the neck, PH, absence of fluid in the stomach and transient alternating filling emptying of a large tubular structure in the fetal neck (proximal esophagus).

Further Reading

Benacerraf BR & Frigoletto FD (1988) Soft tissue nuchal fold in the second trimester fetus: standards for normal measurements compared with those in Down's syndrome. *Am J Obstet Gynecol* 157: 1146.

Bromley B & Benacerraf BR (1995) The resolving nuchal fold in second trimester fetuses not necessarily reassuring. *J Ultrasound Med* 14(3): 253–255.

Hertzberg NS, Bowie JD, Carrol BS et al (1989) Normal sonographic appearances of the fetal neck late in the first trimester. The pseudomembrane. *Radiology* 171: 427.

Sepulveda W, Dezerega V, Horrath E, Aracena M (1999) Prenatal sonographic diagnosis of Aarskog syndrome. *J Ultra Med* 18: 707–710.

Yancy MK, Lasley D & Richards DA (1993) An unusual neck mass in a fetus with Klippel-Trenaunay-Weber syndrome. *J Ultrasound Med* 12: 779–782.

Differential Diagnosis of Neck Webs

- Turner's syndrome
  45X
  Mosaics: X/XX, X/XY, X/XX/XY
  Isochromosome X
  Ring X
  Partial deletion of the X chromosome

- Noonan's syndrome

- Multiple pterygium syndrome

- LEOPARD syndrome

- Aarskog syndrome

Further Reading

Tayabi H & Lachman RS (1996) *Radiology of Syndromes, Metabolic Disorders and Skeletal Dysplasias*, 44th edn. Chicago: Year Book Medical.

5

Fetal Thorax

Fetal breasts

Fetal gynecomastia is a transient phenomenon and may disappear at birth. An ultrasound cross-section through the fetal midthorax will reveal symmetrically enlarged breasts.

Pentalogy of Cantrell

This represents the thoracoabdominal variety of cardiac ectopy (7%). It is characterized by defect of the lower sternum, anterior diaphragmatic hernia, omphalocele, defects in the diaphragm and pericardium and intracardiac defects. Lack of cardiac defects does not fully qualify for this syndrome. Cantrell's pentalogy with ectopia cordis has a very high perinatal mortality rate. Toyama suggested the following classification:

Type I – certain diagnosis contains all 5 defects.
Type II – probable diagnosis with 4 defects (including intracardiac and ventral abdominal wall abnormalities).
Type III – incomplete with various combinations of defects but always including a sternal abnormality. Incomplete expressions of the syndrome are well recognized, e.g no cardiac defects or diaphragmatic defects. US enables diagnosis in the first trimester with state-of-the-art machines. Associations: cystic hygroma, exancephaly, fronto-nasal dysplasia, ABS, cleft

palate and lip, neural tube defects and pericardial effusions.

Ectopia cordis	Cardiac ectopy is classified into five categories depending upon the location of the ectopic heart: cervical, thoracocervical, thoracic, thoracoabdominal and abdominal. It is readily diagnosed as early as the first trimester. Diagnosed as a thoraco-abdominal defect with an extrathoracic pulsating mass, containing Doppler waveforms, typical of intracardiac flow. Doppler helpful in differential diagnosis from cord masses, which have waveforms typical of umbilical artery.
Amniotic bands	Amniotic bands may cause slash defects across the thorax and give rise to various thoracic wall abnormalities including ectopia cordis. Defects are usually atypical and asymmetrical. Identification of a membrane contiguous with such a defect establishes the diagnosis of ABS.
Cystic hygroma	These multiseptate cystic, nuchal masses are usually bilateral, located posterolaterally along the neck, occasionally extending into the upper thorax, upper extremities or mediastinum. Doppler US shows no blood flow within the mass. Cystic hygroma (lymphangioma) in location other than the dorsal nuchal region appear to have little or no known association with aneuploidy. Unlike hemangioma, lymphangiomas do not regress spontaneously.
Limb-body wall complex	This defect may involve the thorax, abdomen or both. Eviscerated organs form a bizarre complex mass entangled with membranes. Defects of the fetal neural axis may be obvious, scoliosis being present in most fetuses. Some authorities are of the belief that LBWC is a complication of ABS.

Chest wall hamartoma
Rare tumor usually diagnosed after birth – benign mesenchymal hamartoma of the chest wall may present with respiratory problems after birth or in early infancy. US: echogenic thoracic wall mass with intrathoracic extension associated with pleural effusion (small) and slightly increased amniotic fluid amount.

Thoracic
myelomeningocele

Hemangioma

Further Reading

Bognoni V, Quartuccio A & Quartuccio A (1999) First-trimester sonographic diagnosis of Cantrell's Pentalogy with exancephaly. *JCU* 27: 276–278.

Cantrell JR, Hellar JA & Ravitsh MM (1958) A syndrome of congenital defects involving the abdominal wall, sternum, diaphragm and heart. *Surgical Gynecology Obstetrics* 107: 602.

Denath FM, Romano W, Solcz M et al (1994) Ultrasonographic findings of exancephaly in Pentalogy of Cantrell: Case report and review of literature. *JCU* 22: 351–354.

Hsieh Y-Y, Lee C-C, Chang C-C et al (1998) Prenatal sonographic diagnosis of Cantrell's pentalogy with cystic hygroma. *JCU* 26: 409–412.

Masuzaki H, Masuzaki M, Ishimaru T & Yamabe T (1996) Chest wall hamartoma diagnosed prenatally using ultrasonography and computed tomography. *JCU* 24: 83–85.

Reichler A & Bronshtein M (1995) Early prenatal diagnosis of axillary cystic hygroma. *J Ultrasound Med* 14: 581–584.

Roberts JA & Sepulveda W (1997) Prenatal sonographic findings associated with lymphangioma of the chest wall. *J Ultra Med* 16: 635–637.

Tongsong T, Wanapirak C, Sirivatanapa P & Wongtrangan S (1999) Prenatal sonographic diagnosis of ectopia cordis. *JCU* 27: 440–445.

Toyama WM (1972) Combined congenital defects of the anterior abdominal wall, sternum, diaphragm, percardium and heart: a case report and review of the syndrome. *Pediatrics* 50: 778.

Fetal Cystic Intrathoracic Masses

Pleural effusions   These appear anechoic and normally conform to the thoracic/diaphragmatic contours.

Teratomas   Anterior mediastinal teratomas are classified into mature and immature types. 17% of mediastinal tumors in children are teratomas of which 1% are immature. Mature teratomas present as large fetal lung tumors with cystic and solid components, PH, hydrops fetalis, pleural effusions and hyperechoic spots with shadowing (calcifications). Immature teratomas form complex masses with multiloculate cystic components associated with PH but may not have calcification or fetal hydrops. In mediastinal teratomas karyotyping is indicated because the prevalence of mediastinal germ cell tumors is 30–50 times higher in Klinefelter syndrome than in the general population.

Bronchogenic cyst   This may be unilocular or multilocular, closely related to the trachea or main bronchus and may communicate with the tracheobronchial tree.

Diaphragmatic hernia   See page 224.

Pericardial cyst   This may be unilocular or multicystic, usually attached to the pericardium overlying the right heart border, or rarely presents at the right costophrenic angle.

Cystic hygroma   Occurs most commonly in association with Turner's syndrome. Usually nuchal, but may rarely extend into the thorax.

Cystic adenomatoid malformation	May be multicystic with evidence of space occupation, or an echogenic mass lesion. Hydrops may occur due to compromise of venous return to the heart. Usually regress during pregnancy. Polyhydramnios may occur. 2% of CCAM are bilateral.
Hemangioma/ lymphangioma	These are rare cystic masses that occupy the mediastinum. Hemangiomas may have a solid component, depending upon the size of vessels involved.
Intralobar sequestration	Cysts are occasionally seen with an intralobar sequestration, which may make differentiation from other cystic intrathoracic masses difficult.
Neuroblastoma	These may be visualized as purely cystic mediastinal masses; however, a complex or solid appearance is not unknown.
Dilated proximal pouch blind esophageal	This has been detected antenatally as a large, purely cystic posterior mediastinal mass.
Mediastinal meningomyelocele/ meningocele	This appears cystic with variable thickness of its wall, which may be associated with vertebral defect; FH and PH may be present.
Cystic dilatation of the bronchus	Massive cystic dilatation involving the left main bronchus has been detected antenatally by sonography.
Enteric/neuroenteric cysts	Usually unilocular, but multilocular posterior mediastinal cysts have been described. Diagnosis is suggested by the position of the cyst adjacent to the bowel and spine. They are often associated with vertebral abnormalities.
Thoraco-abdominal duplication cyst	These cysts should be considered in the differential diagnosis of cystic lesion of both the upper abdomen and thorax, thoracic cysts are usually posterior mediastinal.

Simple lung cyst	These appear as well defined cystic masses, unilocular, surrounded by normal lung.
Prominent pulmonary veins	These may resemble other cystic mediastinal lesions, however, with careful attention to detail, confusion should not arise.
Congenital left ventricular aneurysm	Midline cystic intrathoracic structure in close proximity to the heart, confirmed LV aneurysm by color Doppler.

Further Reading

Bromley B, Parad R, Estroff JA & Benacerraf BR (1995) Fetal lung masses: prenatal course and outcome. *J Ultrasound Med* 14: 927–936.

Markert DJ, Grumbach K & Haney PJ (1996) Thoraco-abdominal duplication cyst; prenatal and postnatal imaging. *J Ultra Med* 15: 333–336.

Rahmani MR, Filler RM & Shuckett B (1995) Bronchogenic cyst occurring in the antenatal period. *J Ultrasound Med* 14: 971–973.

Ray O, Bahado Sing, Romero R et al (1992) Prenatal diagnosis of congenital hiatal hernia. *J Ultrasound Med* 11: 297–300.

Sepulveda W, Drysdale K, Kyle PM et al (1996) Congenital left ventricular aneurysm causing fetal hydrops: prenatal diagnosis with Color Doppler. *J Ultra Med* 15: 327–331.

Wang R-M, Shih J-C & Ko T-M (2000) Prenatal sonographic detection of fetal mediastinal immature teratoma. *J Ultra Med* 19: 289–292.

Fetal Solid Lung Masses

Cystic adenomatoid malformation type III
The cysts are usually so small that they cannot be seen. The multiple interfaces give rise to the impression of an echogenic solid lung mass.

Diaphragmatic hernia
Diaphragmatic hernia is associated with various chromosomal abnormalities including trisomies 13, 18 and 21. The reported incidence of chromosomal anomalies in prenatal series is 20–30%. Other associated abnormalities include CHD (9–23%), neural tube defects (28%) and spinal defects. It is an important feature of Fryn's syndrome. US may reveal polyhydramnios and visualization of abdominal viscera within the thorax. A unilateral pleural effusion may be present. Characteristically, a fluid-filled mass is seen behind the left atrium and ventricle, mediastinal shift is variable. Real-time sonography may reveal bowel peristalsis within the thorax. Solid organs such as the spleen and liver may herniate into the thorax mimicking a solid lung or intrathoracic mass. A clue to liver herniation may be the presence of the gallbladder within the thorax. An associated finding is a reduction in abdominal circumference. Congenital diaphragmatic hernias are unilateral in 97% and usually on the left. Diagnosis of bilateral diaphragmatic hernia is challenging but is possible:

(1) High index of clinical suspicion especially in families with a history of congenital diaphragmatic hernia.
(2) Demonstration of mediastinal shift superiorly and forward position in the chest.
(3) Only mild lateral mediastinal shift.
(4) Careful delineation of hepatic vessels within the thorax can confirm the diagnosis.

Abdominal circumference measurement below the fifth percentile in the second trimester appears to be good predictor as a poor prognosis in fetuses with congenital diaphragmatic hernia.

Lobar sequestration

Lobar sequestration presents as an echogenic lung mass. Cysts can be present in intralobar sequestration, which makes differentiation from type I and II cystic adenomatoid lung difficult.

Extralobar sequestration

Less common than intralobar sequestration. Usually left sided, lying near the diaphragm where it may be confused with a diaphragmatic hernia. Extralobar sequestrations have a good prognosis, unless associated with hydrops and pleural effusions.

Bronchial atresia

US features include enlarged echogenic lung, ascites, hydrops, and abnormalities of the trachea and esophagus.

Congenital lobar emphysema

This must be differentiated from cystic adenomatoid malformation type III. FH is less likely to occur in congenital lobar emphysema.

Chest wall hamartoma

This may be confused with a lung mass. The sonographic features are those of a highly echogenic intrathoracic mass. The mass may be partly calcified and may have densely echogenic areas. The intrathoracic component may be identical to a calcified thoracic neuroblastoma.

Ectopic kidney

Intrathoracic kidney is a rare anomaly, which, if present, usually occurs on the left. The reniform shape, and the absence of the kidney in its normal position, gives away the diagnosis.

Rhabdomyomas

Rhabdomyomas may be cardiac or extra-cardiac. The two varieties are unrelated; the cardiac type are most probably hamartomas. Both types present as solid tumors and are exceedingly rare.

Pericardial tumor

Further Reading

Bromley B, Parad R, Estroff JA & Benacerraf BR (1995) Fetal lung masses: prenatal course and outcome. *J Ultrasound Med.* 14: 927–936.

King SJ, Pilling DW & Walkinshaw S (1995) Fetal echogenic lung lesions: prenatal ultrasound diagnosis and outcome. *Pediatr Radiol* 25: 208–212.

Luet'ic T, Cromblehome TM, Semple JP & D'Alton M (1995) Early prenatal diagnosis of bronchopulmonary sequestration with associated diaphragmatic hernia. *J Ultrasound Med* 14: 533–535.

Maas KL, Feldstein VA, Goldstein RB & Filly RA (1997) Sonographic detection of bilateral fetal chest masses: Report of three cases. *J Ultrasound Med* 16: 647–652.

Mashiach R, Hod M, Friedman S et al (1993) Antenatal ultrasound diagnosis of congenital cystic adenomatoid malformation of the lung: spontaneous resolution in utero. *JCU* 21(7): 453–457.

Paek BW, Danzer E & Machin A (2000) Prenatal diagnosis of bilateral diaphragmatic hernia: Diagnostic pitfalls. *J Ultrasound Med* 19: 495–500.

Teixeira J, Sepulveda W, Hassan J, et al (1997) Abdominal circumference in fetuses with congenital diaphragmatic hernia: correlation with hernia content and pregnancy outcome. *J Ultrasound Med* 16: 407–410.

Multilocular Cystic Intrathoracic Lesions in the Fetus

- **Cystic adenomatoid lung type I and II**
- Bronchogenic cysts
- Lobar sequestration
- Posterior mediastinal enteric cysts
- Neuroenteric cysts
- Cystic hygroma
- Extralobar sequestration
- Esophageal duplication
- Intramural esophageal cysts
- **Diaphragmatic hernia**

Differential Diagnosis of Intrathoracic Echogenic Mass with or without Cystic Component

- CAM
- Sequestration
- Bronchogenic cyst
- Thoracic neuroblastoma
- Tracheal/bronchial atresia
- Congenital lobar emphysema
- Pulmonary AVM

Further Reading

Bromley B, Parad R, Estraff JA & Benacerraf BR (1995) Fetal lung masses: prenatal course and outcome. *J Ultrasound Med* 14: 927–936.

Differential Diagnosis of Cystic Adenomatoid Malformation Type I

- Lobar and extralobar sequestration
- Diaphragmatic hernia
- Cystic teratoma
- Enterogenous or neuroenteric cysts
- Cystic hygroma
- Cystic dilatation of a bronchus
- Simple lung cysts

Differential Diagnosis of Cystic Adenomatoid Malformation Type III

- Lobar sequestration
- Herniated liver
- Congenital lobar emphysema
- Herniated spleen
- Ectopic or herniated kidney

Causes of Fetal Hydrothorax

Fetal pleural effusions may be primary and occur in isolation or as part of FH. Primary effusions are usually chylous and may be unilateral or bilateral.

Immune hydrops	Usually associated with Rh (D) sensitization. Fetal ascites might appear before pleural effusion and skin edema.
Non-immune hydrops	The overall mortality ranges from 50 to 98%. PH is a frequent accompaniment.
Chylothorax	Chylothorax has been seen in association with diffuse congenital lymphangiomatosis, pulmonary lymphangiectasis, congenital lymphedema, diffuse hemangiomas and chylopericardium.
Diaphragmatic hernias	Diaphragmatic hernias are the most frequently encountered intrathoracic masses diagnosed in utero. The bowel, liver, spleen or kidney may be seen. A left-sided hernia usually contains the stomach.
Cystic adenomatoid lung	Lesion usually unilateral but typically involves one lobe or segment. Classified in type I cysts 3–7 cm, type II cysts <1.5 cm and type III cysts so small that they are not discernible on US. Pleural effusion occurs as part of hydrops.
Pena–Shokeir syndrome	Prenatal US may reveal PH, FH, skeletal dysplasias, restricted limb movement, fixed flexion deformity of limbs, absent stomach bubble and kyphosis of the thoracic spine.
Down's syndrome	The syndrome is associated with IUGR, CNS anomalies, cardiac defects, bowel atresias, craniofacial anomalies and limb abnormalities. Ultrasound abnormality is currently only detected routinely in approximately 20–30% of cases.

Turner's syndrome	Prenatal sonographic findings include cystic hygroma, FH, small for gestational age, hiatus hernia and esophageal duplication.
Noonan's syndrome	Associated with limb, rib and vertebral anomalies and lymphatic abnormalities, including pulmonary lymphangiectasis and nuchal cystic hygroma.
Cardiac failure	May be related to structural defect, fetal cardiac arrythmias or cardiomyopathy. Cardiac failure may occur in conjunction with FH.
Fetal hypoalbuminemia	Usually causes bilateral pleural transudates. The low albumin level may be a part of generalized hypoproteinemia secondary to congenital nephrosis (inherited or as a result of CMV infection or renal vein thrombosis).
Cystic hygroma	Fetal pleural effusions have been observed with cystic hygromas, with no associated chromosomal anomalies.
Pulmonary hypoplasia	This may occur as a primary anomaly but is usually secondary to pressure on the developing lung. Several causes have been implicated (see page 235).
Transitory bilateral isolated benign effusions	There are several reports of spontaneous resolution of pleural effusions, particularly those diagnosed in the second or early third trimester.
Intrauterine viral infections	Usually associated with parvovirus infection.
Chest wall hamartoma	Usually small amount.

Further Reading

Laberge JM, Crombleholme TM & Longaker MT (1990) The fetus with pleural effusion. In: Harrison MR, Golbus MS & Filly RA (eds) *The Unborn Patient*, 2nd edn, pp 314–319, Philadelphia: WB Saunders.

Fetal Mediastinal Shift

Diaphragmatic hernia   May contain abdominal viscera, e.g. bowel peristalsis.

Cystic adenomatoid malformation   See page 229.

Diaphragmatic eventration   Abdominal viscera may be seen in the thorax by US. Diagnosis requires visualization of the diaphragm. The abdominal circumference usually remains normal.

Unilateral pleural effusion   US shows anechoic fluid surrounding a lung and displacing the mediastinum. The heart may appear smaller than normal. Large effusions may evert the diaphragm.

Unilateral lung hypoplasia   Search should be made for associated anomalies causing external pressure on the developing lung.

Bronchogenic cyst   These may be intrapulmonary or mediastinal in location and often closely related to the trachea or mainstem bronchi. US appearances may be those of a unilocular or multilocular cyst. There is an association with hemivertebrae.

Neuroenteric cyst   Associated with vertebral abnormalities. Sonography typically shows a unilocular, thin-walled cyst, although multilocular cysts have been described. The diagnosis is suggested by the position of the cyst adjacent to the bowel and spine.

Bronchial atresia   The affected lung may appear normal at midpregnancy; later examinations may show an abnormally echogenic lung with anechoic, dilated, mucus-filled bronchi. Mucus retention and lobar or pulmonary enlargement may cause mediastinal shift.

Esophageal/duplication cyst	Seen as focal fluid collections adjacent to the esophagus. Communication with the esophageal lumen is uncommon and allows the cyst to collapse. Associated anomalies are also uncommon.
Fetal cardiac dextroposition	Fetal cardiac dextroposition and right pulmonary hypoplasia in the absence of an intrathoracic mass are important signs of without intrathoracic right pulmonary hypoplasia, which can be associated with mass significant cardiac and extracardiac abnormalities such as CHD, Scimitar syndrome and left pulmonary artery sling syndrome. Unilateral lung hypoplasia is often associated with pulmonary hypertension, which can complicate the post-clinical state in infants with or without CHD.

Further Reading

Abdullah MM, Lacro RV, Smallborn J et al (2000) Fetal cardiac dextroposition in the absence of an intrathoracic mass: sign of significant right lung hypoplasia. *J Ultrasound Med* 19: 699–676.

Thiagaresch S, Abbott PC, Hogge A et al (1990) Prenatal diagnosis of eventration of the diaphragm. *JCU* 18: 460–449.

Weston MJ, Porter JH, Berry PT et al (1992) Ultrasonographic prenatal diagnosis of upper respiratory tract atresia. *J Ultrasound Med* 11: 673.

Causes of Lung Hypoplasia

Idiopathic

Lung compression syndromes/pulmonary hypoplasia

(a)	**Oligohydramnios**	Severe OH may result in pulmonary hypoplasia, limb-positioning defects and facial anomalies (e.g. Potter's syndrome). OH may be the result of IUGR, renal abnormalities; polycystic renal disease, renal agenesis, renal dysplasia and bladder outlet obstruction.
(b)	**Diaphragmatic hernia**	The most frequently encountered intrathoracic mass diagnosed in utero, often associated with other abnormalities.
(c)	**Thoracic deformity**	e.g. bone dysplasias, rib fractures.
(d)	Premature rupture of membrane	
(e)	**Pleural effusion**	Large effusions may cause the thorax to bulge, with flattening or inversion of the diaphragm.
(f)	Pressure from lung/ mediastinal masses	Cystic adenomatoid lung, bronchogenic cysts, etc.
(g)	**Pressure from abdominal and pelvic masses**	Infantile (autosomal recessive) polycystic kidneys, multicystic dysplastic kidneys, abdominal tumors; pelvic tumors.
(h)	**Cardiac disorders**	Cardiomyopathy
(i)	**Neuromuscular**	Myopathy, skeletal dysplasia
(j)	**Chromosomal anomalies**	Trisomies 21, 18 and 13
(k)	**Idiopathic**	

Further Reading

Fossa S & Esposite V (1994) Fetal pulmonary hypoplasia. *J Perinat Med* 22 (suppl 1): 125–130.

Fox HE & Badalian SS (1994) Ultrasound prediction of fetal pulmonary hypoplasia in pregnancies complicated by oligohydramnios and congenital diaphragmatic hernia: a review. *Am J Perinatol* 11(2): 104–108.

Harstad TW, Twickler DM, Leveno KJ et al (1993) Antepartum prediction of pulmonary hypoplasia: an elusive goal? *Am J Perinatol* 10(1): 8–11.

Hasegawa T, Kamata S, Imura K et al (1990) Use of lung thorax transverse area ratio in the antenatal evaluation of lung hypoplasia in congenital diaphragmatic hernia *JCU* 18: 705.

Sohaey R & Zwiebel WJ (1996) The fetal thorax non-cardiac chest anomalies. *Semin US, CT MRI* 17(1): 34–50.

Diaphragmatic Eventration: Associated Anomalies

- Trisomies 13–15 and 18
- Patent ductus arteriosus
- Aortic stenosis
- Ventricular septal defect
- Hypoplastic aorta
- High-level ectopia
- Turner's syndrome
- Cleft palate and lip
- Bowel volvulus
- Hemivertebra
- Clubfoot
- Hypoplastic ribs

NB Absence of musculature in an area of the diaphragm allows abdominal viscera to bulge into the thorax. The presence of viscera within the thorax may be recognized on ultrasound, but diagnosis of eventration requires visualization of the diaphragm. The abdominal circumference usually remains normal, and the stomach bubble may retain its normal position. Bilateral eventration has been reported with toxoplasma and cytomegalovirus infections.

Further Reading

Thiagaresch S, Abbitt PC, Hoggs A et al (1990) Prenatal diagnosis of eventration of the diaphragm. *JCU* 18: 46–59.

6

Fetal Echocardiography

CHD in parent or sibling	There is a 3–4% incidence of CHD if a sibling is affected. If the mother is affected the risk is up to 12%.
Fetal bradyarrythmias	Atrioventricular block is occasionally associated with endocardial cushion defects, single ventricle and transposition of the great vessels.
Non-immune hydrops	Up to 25% of fetal non-immune hydrops are thought to be related to congenital cardiac anomalies.
Maternal diabetes mellitus	There is a 2% risk of CHD. Poor control of diabetes mellitus in the second and third trimester is associated with hypertrophic cardiomyopathy.
Abnormal karyotype	Especially trisomies 13, 18 and 21.
Exposure to teratogens	The risk of CHD is up to 2% if the mother is exposed to alcohol, amphetamines, anticonvulsants – phenytoin, valproic acid, sex hormones and lithium.
Maternal systemic disorders	These include phenylketonuria, systemic lupus erythematosus and TORCH infections.

Abnormal amniotic fluid volume	
Congenital anomalies known with CHD	Omphalocele, CNS anomalies, abnormal situs, TOF, bowel and esophageal atresias, renal agenesis and diaphragmatic hernia.
Epilepsy	Epileptics have an increased incidence of CHD related both to drug therapy and the underlying disease. Anoxia in early pregnancy is a teratogen.

Fetal Anomalies Associated with Congenital Heart Disease

Central nervous system	Hydrocephalus, microcephaly, agenesis of the corpus callosum, holoprosencephaly, anencephaly, encephalocele.
Gastrointestinal system	GIT atresia, TOF, exomphalos, gastroschisis, diaphragmatic hernia.
Genitourinary system	Renal agenesis, horse-shoe kidney.
Musculoskeletal	Holt–Oram, Fanconi's and Ellis–Van Creveld syndromes, arthrogryposis.
Trisomy 21	Approximately 50% risk of CHD. Associated with endocardial cushion defects, Fallot's tetralogy, VSD.
Trisomy 13/18	Risk of CHD 90-99%. Associated defects are VSD, Fallot's tetralogy, double outflow right ventricle.

Anatomical CheckList of Fetal Four Chamber View

What is the cardiac situs?

Normally the cardiac apex lies on the same side as the left-sided gastric bubble. The right ventricle lies closer to the anterior chest wall than the left. Situs abnormalities are associated with asplenia, polysplenia and complex CHD.

Is the heart normal in size?

The heart occupies approximately one third of the fetal thorax. Standard ratios of external biventricular diameter compared with chest circumference, as obtained by real time and M mode sonography, are available. These ratios may be helpful in predicting cardiomegaly and pulmonary hypoplasia.

Are the two ventricles of approximately equal size?

The two ventricles and atria are of approximately equal size. The muscle mass is also of similar size with the same degree of contractility. The ventricular septum is approximately the same thickness as the ventricular wall.

Is the septum intact?

The flap of foramen ovale should lie in the left atrium. The septum needs careful evaluation as small to moderate VSDs can easily be missed on routine scanning. The use of color flow mapping may allow more accurate diagnosis of VSDs to be made.

What is the position of AV valves?

Of the two AV valves, the tricuspid lies slightly nearer the apex of the heart. The AV valves meet the atrial and ventricular septa to form an offset cross appearance.

Is the endocardium normal?

The moderater band should be visible near the tip of the right ventricle. The valve of the IVC (Eustachian valve) may be seen within the right atrium. In endocardial fibroelastosis, sonography reveals a dilated, poorly contracting heart with diffusely echogenic endocardium.

| Is the myocardium normal? | Cardiomyopathies detected in utero are congestive in type, with a dilated, poorly contracting ventricle and AV valve regurgitation associated with hydrops. Hypertrophic cardiomyopathy has been recognized in association with Noonan's syndrome or poor diabetic control in the third trimester. Rhabdomyomas/rhabdomyosarcoma may cause focal intramural echogenicity. |
| Is the pericardium normal? | A small amount of pericardial fluid is a normal finding but a larger pericardial effusion may be a manifestation of a systemic disorder such as fetal hydrops. |

Further Reading

Brown DL, DiSalvo DN, Frates MC et al (1993) Sonography of the fetal heart: normal variants and pitfalls. *AJR* 160(6): 1251–1255.

McCurdy CM Jr & Reed KL (1993) Basic technique of fetal echocardiography. *Semin US CT MRI* 14: 267–276.

McGahan JP (1991) Sonography of the fetal heart: findings on the four chamber view. *AJR* 156: 5647–5653.

Shultz SM, Pretorius DH & Budovick NE (1994) Four chamber view of the fetal heart: demonstration related to menstrual age. *J Ultrasound Med* 13(4): 285–289.

Sources of Error in Fetal Echocardiography

- Prenatal findings in complex congenital defects tend to underestimate the severity of the abnormalities.
- Mild valve disease may be missed without Doppler because the valves 'look normal.'
- Blood flow velocities may be lower than after birth because of low ventricular pressures present in fetal life, e.g. lack of significant pressure difference across a VSD in utero means that flow through the VSD may not be demonstrable by Doppler.
- Ultrasound resolution is 1–1.5 mm, thus may miss a small VSD.
- Mild aortic coarctation/secundum ASD are 'normal variants' in utero.
- Changes during pregnancy: cardiomyopathies worsen in later weeks and VSD may close in later weeks.
- Aortic isthmus narrowing is a normal feature in utero. It can be distinguished from coarctation because of lack of other recognized features; e.g. left ventricle is normal size not small.
- In complex cardiac defects the main lesion may be recognizable but secondary lesions may be missed.

Fetal Echocardiography: Normal Variants and Artifacts

Four Chamber View

Echogenic foci within ventricles

In the region of the papillary muscles/chordae tendineae small echogenic foci may be seen in the left (up to 20%) or right ventricle (up to 2%) in normal fetuses.

Echogenic mass at edge of myocardium

A small mass, which may at times be very bright and mimic calcification, may be seen at the periphery of ventricular myocardium. This represents artifact and is demonstrated when the imaging plane includes the anterior end of a rib or edge of the sternum.

Prominent Eustachian valve/Chiari's network

These remnants of embryonic valves of the sinus venosus may appear as bright linear structures within the right atrium, and should not be confused with a pathologic process. Chiari's network is sometimes seen as several think echogenic strands within the right atrium; this is usually of no clinical significance, although associated fetal arrythmias have been observed.

Pseudo-VSD

This membranous part of the ventricular septum may occasionally be devoid of echoes mimicking a VSD. This artifact typically occurs when the septum is parallel to the ultrasonic beam; scanning in alternative planes may clarify the situation.

Pseudothickening of tricuspid valve

The parietal band, which represents a band of muscle placed between the tricuspid and pulmonary valves, can be confused with a thickened tricuspid valve.

Pseudo-ASD	The coronary sinus can be identified in the normal fetus. The sinus may become prominent in some forms of anomalous pulmonary venous drainage. The opening of the coronary sinus may be mistaken for lower ASD. Scanning in different anatomical planes should clarify the position.
Pseudopericardial effusion	The peripheral part of the myocardium, which may appear as a hypoechoic rim, may simulate pericardial fluid. A tiny amount of pericardial fluid is normally present and has no pathologic significance.
Pericardial effusion	Small amount of pericardial fluid (<2 mm) is a normal finding although the accuracy of this 2 mm cut-off sign has been questioned. Normal pericardial effusion is generally confined to one part of the pericardium or the level of the AV valve. Pericardial effusion that surrounds the heart is regarded abnormal even when less than 2 mm.

Aortic and Pulmonary Outflow Tracts

Pseudocoarctation	Aortic isthmus narrowing is a normal feature in utero because there is relatively little blood flow through this segment of the aorta. It can be distinguished from coarctation because of the lack of other recognized features, e.g. the left ventricle is normal in size, not small.
Pseudo-overriding of aorta	An overriding aorta occurs when the aortic root is displaced anteriorly so that it arises astride the ventricular septum. There is usually an associated VSD. An overriding aorta can occasionally be simulated. This is an artifact due to a combination of effects. While true overriding is present on several views, pseudo-overriding is usually seen in one place only.

Dilated proximal PA

Slight dilatation of the proximal PA distal to the PV is normally seen and should not be confused with poststenotic dilatation of pulmonary stenosis. True poststenotic dilatation may be confirmed by pulsed or color flow Doppler, which will demonstrate a stenotic jet phenomenon.

Causes of fetal pericardial effusions

- Fetal hydrops – in non-immune hydrops the pericardium is the least frequent location of fluid and pericardial fluid is not universally present.
- Structural heart lesions
- Fetal arrythmias
- Cantrell's pentalogy
- Cardiac tumors
- Bilateral renal anomalies – posterior urethral valves, multicystic dysplasia and renal agenesis.
- Occlusion of the ductus arteriosus due to maternal administration of indomethacin.
- IUGR
- Viral infections – Parvovirus, HIV, CMV and Coxsackie virus.

When a small pericardial effusion is found a maternal antibody screen should be considered. If no associated anomalies and no cause for fetal anemia, viral infection or IUGR, the prognosis is likely to be good.

Further Reading

Bromley B, Lieberman E, Shipp TD et al (1998) Significance of an echogenic intra-cardiac focus in fetuses at high and low risk for aneuploidy. *J Ultrasound Med* 17: 127–131.

Brown DL (1998) Borderline findings in fetal cardiac sonography. *Seminars Ultrasound, CT & MRI* 19: 329–335.

Brown DL, DiSalvo DN, Frates MC et al (1993) Sonography of the fetal heart: normal variants and pitfalls. *AJR* 166: 1251–1256.

Frates MC (1999) Sonography of the normal fetal heart: A practical approach. *AJR* 17: 1363–1370.

Nelson TR, Pretorius DH, Sklorsky M & Hagen-Ansert S (1996) Three dimensional echocardiographic evaluation of fetal heart anatomy and function acquisition, analysis and display. *J Ultrasound Med* 15: 1–9.

Wax JR & Philpot C (1998) Fetal intracardiac foci: Does it matter which ventricle? *J Ultrasound Med* 17: 141–144.

Fetal Cardiac Abnormalities Detectable on Four Chamber View

Absent or small LV

Hypoplastic LV	Often associated with atresias of the mitral and aortic valves. In these cases the heart appears almost to have a single ventricle and outflow tract, although detailed examination may reveal a rudimentary left ventricle and thready aorta.
Mitral atresia	Obstruction/atresia of the mitral valve may occur with an atretic aorta (hypoplastic LV) and with a double outlet RV. In hypoplastic LV syndrome, the aorta is narrow and LV small. The LV cavity may be impossible to demonstrate. In mitral atresia with a double outlet RV there is usually a VSD. The aorta and PA both arise from the RV in a parallel configuration.
Aortic atresia	This may be a part of the hypoplastic left heart syndrome. The aorta is small or absent with a small LV. This is a relatively common condition occurring in up to 20% of cases of CHD detected antenatally. Blood enters the aorta via the ductus arteriosus and thus flow in the ascending aorta may be reversed on color flow Doppler.

Absent or small RV

Hypoplastic RV	This may occur in isolation, or as part of a more complex defect.
Pulmonary atresia	The pulmonary trunk is small or absent. If the ventricular septum is intact the right ventricle is hypertrophied. In early pregnancy the RV may appear enlarged, but in late pregnancy the RV appears small and hypoplastic. Pulmonary atresia may also occur with VSDs and more complex CHD.

Tricuspid atresia — Atresia of the tricuspid valve results in small RV, usually with a VSD. The position of the great arteries is variable and is a major prognostic factor.

Enlarged RV

Coarctation of aorta — Sonographic features include dilatation of the RV and PA which feed the descending aorta via the ductus arteriosus. Narrowing of the aorta may be visible but is difficult to demonstrate.

Tricuspid regurgitation — Regurgitation may be associated with an atretic tricuspid valve or may occur as a part of Ebstein's anomaly.

Pulmonary stenosis — This is likely to cause RV enlargement when the septum is intact.

Pulmonary atresia

Pulmonary regurgitation

Severe IUGR

Enlarged LV

Endocardial fibroelastosis — Sonographic criteria for antenatal diagnosis of fetal endocardial fibroelastosis (FEE) include a dilated LV associated with poor contractility and echogenic foci on the endocardial surface. There are often associated hypoplastic valve(s). FEE may be responsible for signs of CCF/ hydrops and intracavitary thrombus.

Enlarged RA

Ebstein's anomaly

Comprises prolapse of the tricuspid valve into the RV. Tricuspid regurgitation results in right atrial dilatation. When RA dilatation is severe this will cause pulmonary hypoplasia, resulting in poor prognosis. Ultrasonography may also show RV dilatation.

Tricuspid regurgitation

Pulmonary stenosis

This causes RA dilatation when the septum is intact.

Anomalous pulmonary drainage

Drainage is above the diaphragm in 90% of cases. Sonographic features include dilated RA and failure to show normal insertion of pulmonary veins.

Heart failure

This causes dilatation of the right heart chambers and secondary tricuspid regurgitation.

Absent crus

AV canal/endocardial cushion defect

Common AV valve with large combined ASD/VSD. There may be associated conduction defects.

VSD

VSDs are the most common form of CHD found in childhood (20%), although only a quarter of these require surgery. They are not usually evident on antenatal sonography unless part of a complex cardiac malformation.

Single ventricle

This anomaly is usually evident as atria draining into a solitary ventricle, which may mimic a right or left ventricle or represent an indeterminate/intermediate cavity.

Anomalous pulmonary venous drainage

This may be total or partial. Abnormal connection of the pulmonary veins account for 2% of CHD. Abnormal pulmonary venous drainage is classified by the anatomy of the pulmonary venous drainage, which may be:

(1) supracardiac - usually to the left brachio-cephalic veins or less often the SVC;

(2) cardiac - usually to the coronary sinus, occasionally to the right atrium;

(3) infracardiac - to the portal circulation, or the IVC;

(4) mixed - sonographic features include dilated right atrium and failure to show normal insertion of pulmonary veins.

Common pulmonary vein atresia

CPVA is a rare condition in which the pulmonary veins join a blind confluence. The latter has no gross connection either with an atrium or with a systemic vein. A midline enlarged blood vessel may be identified posterior to the heart at the atrial level. It has been suggested that fetal cardiac failure without cardiomegaly should raise the possibility of obstructed pulmonary venous return. Enlarged pulmonary veins are also seen in cases of anomalous pulmonary venous drainage.

Further Reading

Copel JA, Pilu G, Green J et al (1987) Fetal echocardiographic screening for congenital heart disease. The importance of the four chamber view. *Am J Obstet Gynecol* 157: 648–655.

Elliott LP, Anderson RH, Bargeran LM Jr et al (1989) Single ventricle or univentricular heart. In: Adams RH, Emmanouilides GC & Rismenschneider TA (eds) *Heart Disease in Infants, Children and Adolescents,* 4th edn, pp 485–503. Baltimore: Williams & Wilkins.

Ian LD, Crawford DC, Chita SK & Tynan JM (1990) Prenatal screening for congenital heart disease. *BMJ* 292: 1717–1719.

Samuel N, Sirotta L, Bir-Aiv J et al (1988) The ultrasonic appearance of common pulmonary vein atresia in utero. *J Ultrasound Med* 7: 25–28.

Sharland G & Allan L (1990) Detection of congenital abnormalities of the cardiovascular system by ultrasound. In: Chamberlain G (ed.) *Modern Antenatal Care of the Fetus*, p.356, Oxford: Blackwell Scientific.

Sohaey R & Zwiebel WJ (1996) The fetal heart: a practical sonographic approach. *Seminars in US, CT and MRI* 17(1): 15–33.

Tannouri F, Rypens F, Peny M-O et al (1998) Fetal endocardial fibroelastosis: Ultrasonic findings in two cases. *J Ultra Med* 17: 63–66.

Fetal Aortic and Pulmonary Outflow Screening

Most major malformations of the fetal heart may be identified on a four chamber view, however, abnormalities of the outflow tract can easily be missed. The incorporation of outflow tract screening will enhance the sensitivity of diagnosis of anomalies that may be difficult to identify on a four chamber view.

Small Pulmonary Outflow Tract

Tetralogy of Fallot

A large aorta may be the first clue to diagnosis of Fallot's tetralogy. M-mode echocardiography is useful in quantitating the aortic diameter. Doppler may identify a stenotic pulmonary valve as well as showing increased flow through the aorta. The VSD may be difficult to identify on a four chamber view.

Pulmonary atresia

The pulmonary trunk is small or absent and may be difficult to visualize on sonography. It is small in comparison to the aortic root, and may be abnormally sized. If the ventricular septum is intact the RV is hypertrophied. In early pregnancy the RV may appear enlarged but in late pregnancy the RV appears hypoplastic.

Truncus arteriosus

TA is identical in many respects to TF, the only distinguishing feature being that the pulmonary outflow tract is not identified arising from the RV.

Small Aortic Root

Aortic atresia

The aorta is small or absent. The LV is also small. Blood enters the aorta via the ductus arteriosus and thus flow in the ascending aorta may be reversed on color flow Doppler imaging.

Coarctation of the aorta

The aorta appears to be almost half the size of the dilated pulmonary artery. There is right ventricular and right atrial dilatation. M-mode echocardiography may reveal the aortic root diameter at or below the 5th percentile.

Interrupted aortic arch

PA and AA parallel and do not cross at 90°

Transposition

The origins of the great arteries may be reversed, resulting in the aorta arising from the RV, and the pulmonary artery from the LV. There must be communication between these circulations by means of septal defects and the ductus arteriosus to allow survival. Sonographically the aorta arises at 90° to the pulmonary artery but in transposition the aorta arises anterior to the pulmonary artery and runs parallel to it. This abnormality is frequently missed on the four chamber view.

Further Reading

DeVore GR (1985) The prenatal diagnosis of congenital heart disease: a practical approach for the fetal sonographer. *JCU* 13: 229.

DeVore GR, Siassi B & Platt LD (1988) Aortic root dilatation a marker for tetralogy of Fallot. *Am J Obstet Gynecol* 159: 129.

Vergani P, Mariani S, Ghielini A et al (1992) Screening for congenital heart disease with the four chamber view of the heart. *Am J Obstet Gynecol* 167: 1000–1003.

Asymmetry in Fetal Ventricular Size: Right Ventricle Larger than Left Ventricle

Normal
Although the ventricles are usually the same size, in the later stages of pregnancy the right ventricle may be slightly larger than the left.

Coarctation of the aorta
This may range from a minor stenosis to a severe lung atresia. It accounts for 10% of CHD, but only the most severe forms are detected in utero. Marked discrepancy of LV and RV usually means heart anomaly. Mild discrepancy is more problematic, but may be the only sign of co-arctation. The actual narrowing of coarctation may be difficult to identify. The appearance of slight narrowing in the isthmic part of arch can sometimes be seen on US in normal fetuses. Ventricular discrepancy with a slightly small LV compared to RV has only moderate predictive value and sensitivity for coarctation. The potential for false-positive diagnosis is parti-cularly significant in the later part of the third trimester. But it is still a useful sign of coarctation. Other findings in coarctation – abnormal cardiac axis, relatively small aorta at valve level relative to pulmonary artery and predominant left-to-right flow through foramen ovale, hypoplasia of the isthmus and transverse aortic arch, dilatation of RV and pulmonary artery. The aortic lesion is occasionally visible. Coarctation of the aorta is associated with Turner's syndrome, cystic hygroma and fetal hydrops.

Hypoplastic left heart
This is often associated with atresias of mitral and aortic valves. The left ventricle is rudimentary and may be difficult to see. The appearances are those of almost a single ventricle and outflow tract.

Fallot's tetralogy	The aorta is transposed to the right and overlies the ventricular septum. As the aorta overlies the interventricular septum, a VSD is effectively present. Associated features include dextro-position of the aorta, VSD, pulmonary stenosis and right ventricular hypertrophy.
Dysrhythmias	SVT or atrial flutter may result in dilatation of all four chambers or ventricular disproportion. RV enlargement has also been noted with frequent atrial ectopy in the absence of observed tachycardia.
Constriction or occlusion of the ductus arteriosus	May cause RV, right atrium and systemic vein dilatation.
Ventricular dysfunction	RV dysfunction, whatever the cause, may lead to dilatation. Such dysfunction may cause overall cardiac enlargement and secondary tricuspid incompetence.
Tricuspid regurgitation	RV dilatation in tricuspid regurgitation is related to volume overload. Tricuspid regurgitation may be related to twin–twin transfusion syndrome, RV dysfunction, Ebstein's anomaly, cardiomyopathies, anemia, etc.
IUGR	A sizeable proportion of IUGR fetuses have a right ventricle larger than the left.
Left-sided obstructive lesions	Besides coarctation of the aorta and hypoplastic left heart syndrome, mitral stenosis, aortic stenosis/atresia and aortic arch hypoplasia may have a similar effect on ventricular size.
Anomalous pulmonary venous connection	
Miscellaneous conditions	These include parachute mitral valves, some forms of double-outlet right ventricle and atrioventricular canal.

Further Reading

Allan LD, Crawford DC & Tynan MJ (1984) Evaluation of co-arctation of the aorta in intrauterine life. *Br Heart J* 52: 471–473.

Brown DL (1998) Borderline findings in fetal cardiac sonography. *Semin US CT MRI* 19: 329–335.

Marasini M, DeCaro E, Pongiglione G et al (1993), Left heart obstructive disease with ventricular hypoplasia. Changes in the echocardiographic appearances during pregnancy. *JCU 21:* 65–68.

Weil SR & Huhta JC (1993) Sonographic differential diagnosis of fetal cardiac abnormalities. *Semin US CT MRI* 14: 298–317.

Asymmetry in Fetal Ventricular Size: Left Ventricle Larger than Right Ventricle

Hypoplastic right heart — Most authors do not regard a hypoplastic RV as a specific entity. However, this may be considered as a part of pulmonary atresia with an intact ventricular septum or an atretic tricuspid valve in association with a VSD. When the ventricular septum is intact the RV hypoplasia is severe. With an atretic tricuspid valve, the degree of RV hypoplasia depends upon the size of the VSD. These lesions may be progressive in utero.

Pulmonary/tricuspid atresia/stenosis — There may be compensatory enlargement of the LV in tricuspid atresia, and the hypoplastic form of pulmonary atresia with an intact ventricular canal (with a larger inflow to the LV and double inlet LV).

Normal RV functional overload LV — This may be seen occasionally in LV dysfunction in conditions like myocarditis, endocardial fibroelastosis or the dilated form of critical aortic stenosis.

Ebstein's anomaly — In Ebstein's anomaly of the tricuspid valve, the RV may appear small as compared to the normal LV although the atrialized part of RV may be dilated.

Further Reading

Allen LD (1986) Pulmonary atresia in prenatal life. *J Am Coll Cardiol* 8(5): 1131–1136.
Marvin WJ Jr & Mahoney LT (1989) Pulmonary atresia with intact ventricular septum. In: Adams FH, Emmanouilides GC & Riemenschneider TA (eds) *Moss' Heart Disease in Infants, Children and Adolescents,* 4th edn, Baltimore; Williams & Wilkins, pp 338–348.
Well SR & Huhta JC (1993) Sonographic differential diagnosis of fetal cardiac abnormalities. *Semin US CT MRI* 14(4): 298–317.

Masses Related to Fetal Heart

Intracavitary

Papillary muscles/ chordae

These may sometimes be normally prominent and present as small discrete echogenic masses, they should not be confused with pathological tumors.

Moderator band

The moderator band is normally placed with the apex of the RV. Occasionally this band is prominent and mimics a true mass.

Eustachian valve

The valve of IVC (the Eustachian valve) may be see as a bright linear reflector, which is a normal anatomical structure.

Chiari's network

Chiari's network represents remnants of embryonic valves, visualized within the RA as echogenic linear reflectors. They are usually of no significance.

Rhabdomyoma

This is the most common cardiac tumor occurring in the fetus. It is an intramural tumor but may protrude as a pedunculated echogenic mass into the cardiac lumen. They have been diagnosed as early as 16 weeks but are more usually seen at 24 weeks. Associated with tuberous sclerosis.

Fibroma

These tumors lie within the cardiac wall but may present as echogenic pedunculated intra-cavitary masses. Arrythmias and sudden death are common.

Hamartoma

This tumor has been reported as an intracavitary mass lesion in a newborn who presented with an arrhythmia.

Hemangioma

An intra-atrial hemangioma has been identified retrospectively in a fetus, associated with hydrops.

Intramural

Rhabdomyoma

This is usually sessile and arises from the myocardium. The tumor is usually of the same echogenicity as normal myocardium but can be highly echogenic. Fetal arrythmias are common. Larger masses may obstruct blood flow. They may be associated with tuberous sclerosis.

Fibromas

Fibromas are rare cardiac mass lesions. They may be solitary or multiple and may lie within the cardiac wall or be pedunculated, protruding into the cardiac cavity. The appearances may therefore be identical to rhabdomyomas.

Bronchogenic cysts

These lung/mediastinal masses may rarely occur within the myocardium and may even project into the ventricle or pericardial space. They have been reported in the newborn but not the fetus and do not usually cause hemo-dynamic disturbance.

Mesothelioma of atrioventricular node

This is an extremely rare intramural mass lesion which may present with cardiac arrhythmia.

Intrapericardial

Teratoma

Teratoma is the second most commonly occurring cardiac tumor in the fetus. It arises from the pericardium and may be cystic and pedunculated and may calcify. It is often associated with a pericardial effusion and may cause cardiac tamponade. Hydrops may also occur, particularly if masses obstruct the right ventricular inflow.

Morgagni's hernia

Rarely the pericardium may be continuous with the peritoneum via the foramen of Morgagni. Bowel or liver may therefore herniate into the pericardium and mimic a teratoma.

Peripericardial

Pericardial cyst	The majority of these cysts are present at the right cardiophrenic angle, although some have been reported on the left. The cysts are usually attached to the pericardium, and vary in size from one to several centimeters. They are usually filled with clear fluid. Larger cysts may project into the anterior or posterior mediastinum.
Teratoma	This is usually a pericardial tumor but may project into the pericardial space. When cystic they may be indistinguishable from pericardial cysts. They may calcify and are associated with pericardial effusions, cardiac tamponade and fetal hydrops.

Further Reading

Brown DL, DiSalvo DN, Frates MC et al (1993) Sonography of the fetal heart. Normal variants and pitfalls. *AJR* 166: 1251–1255.

Brown DL, Roberts DJ & Miller WA (1994) Left ventricular echogenic focus in the fetal heart: pathologic correlation. *J Ultrasound Med* 13(8): 613–616.

Coates TL & McGahan JP (1994) Fetal rhabdomyomas presenting as diffuse myocardial thickening. *J Ultrasound Med* 13: 281–283.

de Bustamante TD, Azpeitia J, Miralles M et al (2000) Prenatal sonographic detection of pericardial teratoma. *J Ultra Med* 28: 194–198.

Weil SR & Huhta JC (1993) Sonographic differential diagnosis of fetal cardiac abnormalities. *Semin US CT MRI* 14: 289–317.

Fetal Acardia

Acardia

Acardia occurs in 1% of monozygote twin pregnancies. The pregnancy in which this anomaly occurs will have a single placenta, but there may be one or two amnions. When a monochorionic twin pregnancy has only one amnion, acardia risk is six times as great as when two amnions are present. US reveals absent cardiac motion in the abnormal twin.

Types of Acardia

Acardius acephalus

This is the most common type of acardia (60–75%). There is no head. The abdomen is developed but there are no thoracic organs. The upper extremities may or may not be present. PH may be present with functioning kidneys.

Acardius anceps

The head and face are partially developed. The body and extremities are developed but the heart is absent. There is increased amount of soft tissue with or without cystic areas. PH may be present if the fetus has functioning non-obstructed kidneys.

Acardius amorphous

A formless blob containing all tissue types but no recognizable organs. This differs from a teratoma only in its attachment to an umbilical cord.

Acardius acormus

There is a head but no body. This is the rarest type.

Further Reading

Acton CM & Woodward CS (1993) Acardiac twins. *Australas Radiol* 37: 389–391.

Al-Malt A, Ashmead G, Mann L et al (1991) Color-flow and Doppler velocimetry in prenatal diagnosis of acardiac triplet. *J Ultrasound Med* 10: 341–345.

Landy HJ, Larsen JW, Schaen M et al (1989) Acardiac fetus in a triplet pregnancy. *Teratology* 37: 1.

Moore TR, Gale S & Benirschke K (1990) Prenatal outcome of forty-nine pregnancies complicated by acardiac twinning. *Am J Obstet Gynecol* 163: 907.

Pretoruis DH, Leopold GR, Moore TR et al (1988) Acardiac twin report of Doppler sonography. *J Ultrasound Med* 7: 419.

Rydert J, Holmgren G & Gigurd J (1984) Intra-uterine diagnosis of an acardiac monster. *Acta Obstet Gynecol Scand* 63: 569.

Wexler S, Baruch A, Ekstein N et al (1985) An acardiac acephalic anomaly detected on sonography. *Acta Obstet Gynecol Scand* 674: 93.

Fetal Arrhythmias

Premature atrial beats	Premature atrial beats are common, accounting for 60–70% of fetal arrhythmias. They may rarely progress to SVT.
Sinus tachycardia	The normal fetal heart rate is 120–170/min. Sinus tachycardia occurs with beats above 170/min. Fetal tachycardia may be secondary to maternal disease, e.g. maternal pyrexia or thyrotoxicosis.
Supraventricular tachycardia	SVT accounts for up to 15% of arrhythmias. Heart rates of 200–300/min are recorded, which, if they persist, may cause fetal heart ± fetal hydrops. Ten per cent have underlying CHD. Maternal treatment is with digoxin or flecainide.
Atrial flutter	This results in cardiac contractions of up to 400/min. Not all atrial beats are conducted. The rapid heart rate may result in heart failure, causing hydrops. Maternal treatment with digoxin may be effective. Rarely atrial flutter may be associated with CHD and intracardiac tumors.
Atrial fibrillation	This has been recognized but is extremely rare.
Ventricular tachycardia	This has been recorded but appears to be extremely rare.
Sinus bradycardia	Sinus bradycardia is uncommon but may be a sign of fetal distress, particularly in late pregnancy, in which case the fetus should be evaluated for other signs of fetal compromise.

Atrial bigeminy

Blocked premature atrial contraction not conducted to the ventricles resulting in dropped beats. A common benign arrhythmia which usually resolves spontaneously but may progress to SVT. The heart rate is usually below 110/min.

Atrioventricular block

Complete AV block produces a heart rate of 40–80/min. The incidence of complete heart block is significantly higher in fetuses with maternal connective tissue disease. Fetal hydrops may occur in the third trimester. US reveals a slow ventricular rate with lack of correlation with atrial activity. Maternal anti-Rho antibodies should be assessed.

NB   M-mode echocardiography is a useful means of demonstrating the cause of a rhythm disturbance as it can simultaneously display atrial and ventricular motion. An M-mode section through the left ventricle shows ventricular wall motion and also the FAC wave of the mitral valve trace, i.e. atrial systole. Doppler can be used in a similar manner. Reviewing images of mechanical events in this way is less precise than ECG but the fetal ECG has almost no P waves, which can make the exact timing of atrial systole difficult to determine.

Further Reading

DeVore GR, Biassi B & Platt LD (1990) The fetus with cardiac arrhythmias. In: Harrison MR, Golbus MS & Filly RA (eds) *The Unborn Patient,* 2nd edn, pp 249–263, Philadelphia: WB Saunders.

Doubilet PM & Benson CB (1995) Embryonic heart rate in the early first trimester. What rate is normal? *J Ultrasound Med* 14:431–434

Fyfe DA, Meyer KB & Case CL (1993) Sonographic assessment of fetal cardiac arrhythmias. *Semin US CT MRI* 14: 286–297.

7

Fetal Abdomen and Pelvis

Anterior External Masses of the Fetal Abdomen

Physiological bowel herniation

Physiological herniation occurs at 10–13 weeks. The best discriminating method for differentiating this from an omphalocele is to perform a repeat sonogram after 15 weeks menstrual age. A large defect with liver exteriorized indicates an omphalocele at any gestation.

Omphalocele

Omphalocele is herniation of a variable amount of abdominal viscera through a defect (2–10 cm) at the base of the umbilical cord. A membrane covers the herniation, differentiating it from gastroschisis, and the umbilical vessel inserts into the apex. There is frequent association of liver herniation, ascites, cardiac defects and chromosomal anomalies. Association with holoprosencephaly and limb anomalies is occasional. High incidence of chromosomal abnormality – approximately one third. Prognosis is related to the karyotype, associated abnormalities and contents of the omphalocele.

Umbilical hernia	Umbilical hernia is due to a defect in the linea alba; the protruding bowel is covered by subcutaneous tissues and skin. Umbilical hernia is common in the first months in 20% of African-American infants and 3% of white neonates. It is frequent in premature infants >5% of those weighing less than 1500 grams. US: prominent bulge of the anterior abdominal wall which may contain omentum/bowel, which may protrude into the umbilical cord. Amniotic fluid AFP may be elevated when bowel herniates into the umbilical cord.
Gastroschisis	Gastroschisis results from herniation/ evisceration of bowel and occasionally the bladder and adnexa into the amniotic cavity through a small defect (2–5 cm) in the right paraumbilical region. There is no covering membrane. It is thought to result from a vascular event to the omphalomesenteric artery. Vascular compromise may occur from volvulus and may result in obstruction, ischemia and atresia. Bowel wall thickening occurs. Not associated with other abnormalities and the chromosomes are normal. Prognosis good. The presence of liver and spleen herniation has been reported to modify the prognosis and work-up. The pancreas, stomach, bladder, uterus, ovaries and the fallopian tubes may also herniate.
Amniotic bands	ABS is a common cause of abdominal wall defect. Involvement of the abdominal wall may produce appearances similar to gastroschisis. However, an atypical location of the abdominal wall defect should suggest the diagnosis of ABS. Membranes contiguous with such a defect may be identified.

Extrophy of bladder	Sonographically bladder extrophy may present as an external, well defined, solid or complex mass immediately superior to the fetal genitalia. Prolonged and repeated scans will fail to reveal the fetal bladder. The renal collecting system and ureters need not be dilated, whereas unilateral or horseshoe kidneys may be found. Uterine and adnexal anomalies are relatively frequent. The pubis is abnormally wide and the umbilical cord insertion may be abnormal.
Thoracoabdominal pentalogy of Cantrell	Ectopia cordis associated with a ventral wall defect should prompt the diagnosis of PC. The syndrome is often associated with other anomalies.
Cloacal extrophy	This consists of a low omphalocele, bladder or cloacal extrophy and frequently other caudal anomalies, including meningomyelocele, anal atresia and lower limb anomalies. Most affected fetuses have a single umbilical artery. US: low anterior abdominal mass below umbilical cord associated with an absent urinary bladder.
Limb-body wall complex	LBWC is a lethal condition with severe anterior abdominal wall defect, the defect placed laterally, which involves the umbilical cord insertion size. The abdominal contents lie outside within a sac of amnion and mesoderm. There is a frequent association with CHD, cranial anomalies (encephalocele), limb abnormalities and scoliosis. Chromosomal defects are not usually present.
Multiple cavernous hemangiomas	These are most frequently found over the lower body and are often associated with Klippel–Trenaunay–Weber syndrome, which is diagnosed in the presence of multiple surface masses producing limb hypertrophy. Hydrops may occur.

Further Reading

Abu-Yousel MM, Wray AB, Williamson RA et al (1987) Antenatal ultrasound diagnoses of variant of pentalogy of Cantrell. *J Ultrasound Med* 6: 535.

Emanuel PG, Garcia GI & Angtuaco TL (1995) Prenatal detection of anterior abdominal wall defects with US. *Radiographics* 15(3): 517-530.

Gray DL, Maretin CM, Crane JP et al (1989) Differential diagnoses of first trimester ventral wall defects. *J Ultrasound Med* 8: 255-258.

Hortijin CG, Philip AG, Anderson GG et al (1981) The in utero-ultrasonographic appearances of Klippel-Trenaunay-Weber syndrome. *Am J Obstet Gynecol* 129: 972-974.

Maynor CH, Herzbert GS & Kliewer MA (1995) Antenatal ultrasonographic diagnosis of abdominal wall hemangioma: potential to stimulate ventral abdominal wall defects. *J Ultrasound Med* 14: 317-319.

Nyberg DA (1989) Chromosomal abnormalities in fetuses with omphalocele: significance of omphalocele: significance of omphalocele contents. *J Ultra Med* 8: 229.

Pattern RM, Van Allen M, Mack LA et al (1986) Limb body wall complex: in utero sonographic diagnosis of a complicated fetus malformation. *AJR* 146: 1019-1024.

Richards DS, Kays DW (1998) Prenatal ultrasonographic diagnosis of a simple umbilical hernia. *J Ultra Med* 17: 265-267.

Shalev E, Eliyahu S, Battino S & Weiner E (1995) First trimester transvaginal sonographic diagnosis of body stalk anatomy. *J Ultrasound Med* 14: 641-642.

Snijders RJM, Brizot ML, Faria M & Nicolaides KH (1995) Fetal exomphalos at 11 to 14 weeks of gestation. *J Ultrasound Med* 14: 569-574.

Tannouri F, Avni EF, Lingier P et al (1998) Prenatal diagnosis of atypical gastroschisis. *J Ultra Med* 17: 177-180.

Absent or Small Fetal Stomach

A fluid-filled stomach is nearly always seen in normal fetuses in the second and third trimester. An absent fetal stomach after 18 weeks gestation is associated with a guarded prognosis with abnormal outcome in 48–100%. A small fetal stomach has also been reported to have an abnormal outcome in 52% of fetuses. The ultimate prognosis depends on associated abnormalities. A small fetal stomach is difficult to assess although normograms of fetal stomach size have been published, the validity of stomach measurements has been questioned because of the dynamic nature of the fetal stomach filling and emptying. In one study when a small fetal stomach was assessed; the stomach was regarded as small if during a 45-minute examination it was difficult to visualize and revealed a small fluid-filled stomach in the left upper quadrant. An abnormal outcome is related to amniotic fluid volume, the poorest prognosis occurs when a small or absent stomach is related to associated OH (88%) or PH (84%). 28% have abnormal karyotype and 15% have esophageal atresia.

Normal (transient)	The stomach is visualized in virtually all fetuses from 20 weeks onwards. After contraction the stomach may be transiently absent.
Esophageal atresia	With esophageal atresia, the stomach remains empty except where there is associated TOF.
VACTERAL	TOF is associated with complex anomalies, including vertebral, anal, cardiac, renal and limb abnormalities (VACTERAL). The absence of stomach in the presence of PH should raise the possibility of esophageal atresia.
Cleft lip and palate	Related to inability or inefficient swallowing of amniotic fluid.
Neck masses	Any neck or thoracic mass can give rise to mechanical obstruction of swallowing reflex.
Oligohydramnios	Related to reduction of amniotic fluid available to the fetus to swallow.

Distressed fetus	Poorly filled stomach has been observed in the severely distressed fetus, e.g. in non-immune hydrops or severe IUGR.
Congenital diaphragmatic hernia (abnormally sited stomach)	In a left-sided hernia the stomach is often displaced into the thorax with small and large bowel. Mediastinal shift is usually apparent. Thirty per cent associated structural defect – cardiac, renal, skeletal most commonly; 30% associated chromosomal defect. Approximately 70% loss rate.
Neurological obstruction	Pena Shokier syndrome and arthrogryposis.

Further Reading

Goldstein RB & Callen PW (1994) Ultrasound evaluation of the fetal thorax and abdomen. In: Callen PW (ed.). *Ultrasonography in Obstetrics and Gynecology*, 3rd edn, pp 333–369. Philadelphia: WB Saunders.

McKenna KM, Goldstein RB & Stringer MD (1995) Small or absent fetal stomach. *Radiology* 197(3): 729–733.

Gastric Filling Defects

Pseudomasses

    (a)   Caused by peristaltic wave in gastric wall.

    (b)   Most probably related to aggregates of cellular debris from swallowed amniotic fluid, and vernix near the end of pregnancy. These masses are not constant and may not be found on subsequent scanning.

Swallowed meconium

Echogenic gastric intraluminal masses changing position with fetal movement.

Swallowed blood

Fetal 'Double Bubble' Sign

Duodenal atresia

This lesion is usually associated with PH and a 'double bubble' sign as a result of a dilated stomach and proximal duodenum. The appearances are those of two communicating cystic masses in the upper abdomen. Thirty per cent association with trisomy 21.

Duodenal stenosis

Signs in duodenal stenosis are variable and may not be present in utero. Normally the fetal duodenum is non-distended. Persistent duodenal fluid-filled distention may be an early sign of duodenal obstruction.

Jejunal atresia

PH is a feature of most upper bowel obstruction, whatever the cause. In common with other upper GI obstructions the presence of dilated loops of bowel may be seen. Jejunal atresia may give rise to a 'triple bubble' sign. The typical appearances are those of proximal small bowel dilatation appearing as multilocular sonolucent masses. There may be a single fluid-filled bubble in the abdomen, demonstrating peristaltic movement of small particles in the fluid-filled lesion, but no dilatation in other parts of the intestine.

Annular pancreas

This is a rare congenital anomaly that may give rise to upper GI obstruction and potentially give rise to a 'double bubble' sign.

Other causes of upper GIT obstruction

These include congenital bands, internal hernias, volvulus, cystic fibrosis and meconium ileus.

Normal variant

A normal stomach divided by a prominent wave of peristalsis may superficially resemble a 'double bubble' but this is likely to be a transient phenomenon. Meconium may acquire an anechoic state and thus meconium in the transverse colon close to the stomach may mimic a 'double bubble' when scanning in the transverse plane. Care should be taken not to misinterpret a normal gallbladder adjacent to the stomach as 'double bubble.'

Normal stomach with adjacent fluid-filled structure

A normal fluid-filled stomach with an adjacent fluid-filled cystic mass may resemble a 'double bubble.' These cystic lesions include renal, choledochal, hepatic, adrenal, mesenteric, duplication and retroperitoneal cysts and hydronephrosis.

Congenital duplication of stomach

Duplication cysts may occur at any point in the GIT and may be multiple. The stomach is less frequently affected than other regions. A cystic mass in the right upper quadrant has been reported: it proved to be a gastric duplication cyst.

Causes of Fetal Gastric Dilatation Associated with Hydramnios

- Pyloric atresia
- Preantral web
- Pyloric stenosis
- Non-hypertrophic pyloric stenosis associated with intestinal malrotation
- Duodenal and proximal jejunal atresia (50% associated with PH)
- Rarely seen in the presence of obstruction of the distal ileum and colon

Echogenic fetal bowel

Various grading systems have been proposed to identify echogenic bowel. The bowel is classified as moderately/markedly echogenic when its echogenicity is close that of bone.

Grade I = bowel > echogenic than liver. Grade II = > echogenic than bone. Causes:

- Normal variant
- Meconium ileus
- Cystic fibrosis
- Chromosomal abnormality – particularly trisomy 21
- IUGR
- Intrauterine infections
- Intra-amniotic bleeding
- Obstructive GIT disease
- Bowel ischemia

Dilated fetal bowel

The small bowel can be identified in the second trimester and normally measures on the average 1.2 mm (range 1.0–1.5 mm) before 30 weeks gestation. The small can be identified in only 30% of fetuses after 34 weeks. In fetuses with bowel lumen >2 mm, low or absent AF disaccharidase activity is associated with intestinal obstruction. Causes of dilated fetal bowel:

- Large or small bowel atresia
- Malrotation with intestinal duplication
- Meconium ileus
- Meconium plug syndrome
- Echogenic dilated bowel loops (EBDL): this is a new entity most likely related to temporary obstruction from mesenteric ischemia, leading to transient obstruction. Fetuses with isolated EBDL have a good prognosis, while fetuses with a complex form of EDBL depends upon the severity of related abnormality.
- Congenital small bowel syndrome: Fatal but rare condition, a few familial cases reported associated with malrotation. Unlike the various conditions of acquired short-bowel syndrome it is characterized by severe intestinal dysmotility. US: Delayed return of midgut to the abdominal cavity, dilated loops bowel and PH.

Differential diagnosis of delayed midgut return

Normally as the midgut elongates by the 5th gestation week it forms a loop that extends into the umbilical coelom. The intestine usually returns to the abdominal cavity by the 10th week gestation. Causes of delayed midgut return:

- Congenital small bowel syndrome
- Intestinal obstruction
- Volvulus of the small bowel

Further Reading

Aviram R, Erez I, Dolfin TZ et al (1998) Congenital short-bowel syndrome: Prenatal sonographic findings of fetal anomaly. *JCU* 26: 106–108.

Bidwell JK & Nelson A (1986) Prenatal ultrasonic diagnosis of congenital duplication of the stomach. *J Ultrasound Med* 5: 589–591.

Bonin B, Gruslin A, Simpson NAB et al (1998) Second trimester prenatal diagnosis of congenital gastric outlet obstruction. *J Ultra Med* 17: 403–406.

Boychuk RB, Lyons EA & Goodhand TK (1978) Duodenal atresia diagnosed by ultrasound. *Radiology* 127: 500.

Feltman D, McQuon D, Kanchanapoom V et al (1980) 'Apple peel' atresia of the small bowel prenatal diagnosis of the obstruction by ultrasound. *Pediatr Radiol* 9: 118–119.

Font GE & Salari M (1998) Prenatal diagnosis of bowel obstruction, initially manifested as isolated hyperechoic bowel. *J Ultra Med* 17: 721–723

Grigon A, Dubois J, Ouellet M-C et al (1997) Echogenic dilated bowel loops before 21 weeks gestation: A new entity. *AJR* 168: 833–837.

Houlton MCC, Sutton M & Aitken J (1974) Antenatal diagnosis of duodenal atresia. *J Obstet Gynaecol Br Commonwealth* 81: 810–821.

Kubota A, Nakayama T, Yonekura T et al (2000) Congenital ileal atresia presenting as a single cyst-like lesion on prenatal sonography. *JCU* 28: 206–208.

Levine D, Goldstein RB, Cadrin C (1998) Distension of the fetal duodenum: abnormal find? *J Ultra Med* 17: 213–215.

Nelson LH, Clarke CE, Fishburn JI et al (1982) Value of serial sonography in the in utero detection of duodenal atresia. *Obstet Gynecol* 59: 657–660.

Nikapota ULB & Loman C (1979) Grey scale sonographic demonstration of fetal small bowel atresia. *JCU* 7: 307–310.

Parulekar SG (1991) Sonography of normal fetal bowel. *J Ultrasound Med* 10: 211–220.

Quimette MV & Bree R (1984) Sonography of pelvo-abdominal cystic masses in children and adolescents. *J Ultrasound Med* 3: 149.

Samuel N, Dicker D, Feldberg D et al (1984) Ultrasound diagnosis and management of fetal intestinal obstruction and volvulus in utero. *J Perinat Med* 12: 333–337.

Stickler K, Vang R & Maklad N (1998) Echogenic fetal bowel and calcified meconium in a fetus with trisomy 21. *J Ultra Med* 17: 591–593.

Cystic Fetal Abdominal Masses

Gastrointestinal Tract

Normal fluid filled bowel

Cystic fibrosis/meconium pseudocyst/peritonitis

Dilated loops of bowel due to obstruction

Bowel atresias/stenoses

Volvulus

Mesenteric/omental cyst

Hirschsprung's disease

Duplications	Gastric duplication cysts present as anechoic lesions, the wall of the cyst may show an inner hyperechoic layer representing the mucosa and the hypoechoic outer layer representing the muscular layer. Occasionally the cyst may appear echogenic due to hemorrhage or inspissated material within the cyst.

Liver, Pancreas and Spleen

Choledochal cysts	Choledochal cyst is a cystic dilatation of the biliary system.

Mesenchymal hamartoma

Liver hemangioma

Hepatic cysts

Pancreatic cysts/pseudocyst	Congenital pancreatic cysts may be unilocular or multilocular associated with PH and hydrops. 63% are associated with more complex syndromes such as Beckwith–Wiedemann syndrome, skeletal dysplasia and hemihypertrophy.
Splenic cyst	Splenic cysts may change size and shape with advancing menstrual age.
Omphalomesenteric duct cyst	Various portions of omphalomesenteric duct may persist, giving rise to Meckel's diverticulum, intra-abdominal omphalomesenteric cyst, anomalies of the umbilicus such as fistulas, polyps or cysts of the umbilical cord, or a combination of these lesions. Cysts of the umbilical cord are usually small, but may be as large as 6 cm in diameter. These cysts are situated close to the abdominal wall. There is usually no blood flow through them.
Vesicoallantoic abdominal defect	Failure of the allantoic cavity to obliterate results in vesicoallantoic communication between the bladder and umbilicus that may fall into one of four types: (1) patent urachus; (2) vesicourachal diverticulum; (3) umbilical cyst and sinus; (4) alternating urachal sinus. There is a common association with other genitourinary anomalies, urethral obstruction being the most common. Sonographically, continuity of an anterior abdominal wall mass with fetal bladder establishes the diagnosis of a vesicoallantoic cyst prenatally.

Genitourinary

Hydronephrosis

Distended urinary bladder

Rental cysts

Cystic renal dysplasia

Urinoma

Ovarian cyst/neoplasm	These are not uncommon. Cysts may be simple or theca lutein cysts. Fetal theca lutein cysts are associated with maternal diabetes mellitus. Cysts may be unilocular or multiseptate. This is the most frequent cause of cystic lower abdominal mass in the female fetus. In utero torsion can occur.
Wolffian duct cyst	Wolffian duct cysts arise as a result of cystic distension of imperfectly obliterated regions of the duct. They are only seen in female fetuses. Gartner's duct (the terminal paravaginal portion of the Wolffian duct) is the most common site of cyst formation. The cysts are usually small, unilocular, placed between the kidneys and bladder. Diagnosis has been made antenatally at 33 weeks, when three communicating cysts were demonstrated.
Cloacal dysgenesis	This is related to incomplete partitioning of the common cloaca and may give rise to septate pelvic mass or multiple thin-walled cysts of varying sizes. There is association with other anomalies of the genitourinary tract, respiratory tract, CVS, skeletal system and anencephaly.
Hydrocolpos/ hydrometrocolpos	A cystic mass arising from the pelvis. Duplication of the vagina and uterus may result in a multiseptate configuration. Associated anomalies include hydronephrosis, bowel obstruction due to extrinsic compression, TOF, esophageal and duodenal atresias and mal-rotation. May cause PH, but OH may occur with urinary tract obstruction.

Retroperitoneum

Adrenal cysts/hemorrhage

Retroperitoneal cysts

Retroperitoneal cysts are similar so other abdominal cysts of mesenteric and bowel origin, and frequently cannot be differentiated from these on US. They usually lie in the midabdomen.

Lymphangioma

Like hemangiomas it is difficult to be certain as to whether lymphangiomas are true tumors i.e. hamartomas or lymphangiectasias (benign). The majority occur in the fetal neck – cystic hygroma (75%) and the axilla (20%). Other sites include face, tongue, abdomen, mediastinum, abdominal viscera and bone (5%). Abdominal lymphangiomas are rare. US: Hypoechoic mass with different levels of attenuation (depending on the nature of contained fluid i.e. serum, chylous, etc.) of varying sizes, well-defined unilocular or multilocular with fine septations. An intracystic hemorrhage may modify the appearance.

Masses Related to Spine/Sacrum

Sacrococcygeal cyst/teratoma

Anterior meningocele

Umbilical Vein Masses

Dilated umbilical vein

Umbilical vein varices

Hypoechoic Meconium

Meconium distended rectum

Meconium in sigmoid colon

Further Reading

Cornstock CH (1988) Fetal masses ultrasound diagnosis and evaluation. *Ultrasound Q* 6: 229–256.

Devesa R, Munoz A, Torrents M, Carrera JM (1997) Prenatal ultrasonographic findings of intra-abdominal cystic lymphangioma. *JCU* 25: 330–332.

Donnerfield AE, Mannuli MT, Templeton JM et al (1989) Prenatal sonographic diagnosis of a vesico-allantoic abdominal defect. *J Ultrasound Med* 8: 43–45.

Fink IJ & Filly RA (1983) Omphalocele associated with umbilical cord allantoic cysts: Sonographic evaluation in utero. *Radiology* 149: 473.

Gallagher DM, Leiman S & Hux CH (1993) In utero diagnosis of a portal vein aneurysm. *JCU* 21: 147–151.

Hill LM (1988) Sonographic detection of fetal gastro-intestinal anomalies. *Ultrasound Q* 6: 35–67.

Hill SJ & Hirsch JN (1988) Sonographic detection of fetal hydrometrocolpos. *J Ultrasound Med* 4: 323.

Kapor R, Sala MM & Mandal AK (1989) Antenatal sonographic detection of Wolffian duct cysts. *JCU* 17: 515–517.

Lichman JP & Miller EI (1988) Prenatal ultrasonic diagnosis of splenic cyst. *J Ultrasound Med* 7: 637–638.

McCalla CO, Lajinian S, DeSouza D & Rottem S (1995) Natural history of antenatal omphalomesenteric duct cyst. *J Ultrasound Med* 14: 639–640.

Macken MB, Wright JR, Lau H et al (2000) Prenatal sonographic detection of congenital hepatic cyst in the third trimester after normal second trimester sonographic examination. *JCU*: 28 307–310.

Nowell RM, Jaffe R, Sanko JR and Hulbert WC (1995) Changing ultrasonographic appearances of a vesicoallantoic abdominal wall defect. *JCU* 23:391–394.

Okada M, Hata T, Ariyuki Y et al (1995) Fetal splenic cyst: change in size and shape with advancing menstrual age. *JCU* 23: 204–206.

Ozman MN, Ondergolu L, Cifli AO et al (1997) Prenatal diagnosis of gastric duplication cyst. *J Ultra Med* 16: 219–222.

Parulekar SG (1991) Sonography of normal fetal bowel. *J Ultrasound Med* 10: 211–220.

Rosenberg JC, Chervenak FA, Walker BA et al (1986) Antenatal sonographic appearances of omphalo-mesenteric duct cyst. *J Ultrasound Med* 5: 719–720.

Sach L, Fourcroy JL, Wenzel DJ et al (1992) Prenatal detection of umbilical cord allantoic cyst. *Radiology* 145: 445.

Sepulveda W, Carsten E, Sanchez J, Cutierrez J (2000) Prenatal diagnosis of congenital pancreatic cyst: case report and review of literature. *J Ultra Med* 19: 349–352.

Song S & Ding J (1995) Prenatal ultrasonic findings of Wolffian duct cyst. *JCU* 23: 333 [letter].

Weston MJ & Andrews H (1991) In utero aspiration of a sacrococcygeal cyst. *Clin Radiol* 44:119–120.

Differential Diagnosis of Sacrococcygeal Teratoma

- Bladder outlet obstruction
- Meningomyelocele
- Ovarian teratomas
- Neuroblastoma
- Retrorectal hamartoma
- Intracanalicular epidermoid tumors
- Dermal sinus stalk ascending towards the conus medullaris
- Hydromelia
- Lipoma
- Extrarenal Wilms' tumor

Fetal Pelvic Masses

- Ovarian cyst/tumor
- Dilated bowel
- Distal rectum
- Mesenteric cyst
- Urachal cyst
- Sacrococcygeal teratoma
- Bowel duplication cyst
- Wolffian duct cyst
- Meconium pseudocyst
- Hydrometrocolpos
- Anterior meningocele
- Bowel perforation with loculated ascites

Differential Diagnosis of a Fetal Abdominal Multilocular Cystic Mass

Multicystic dysplastic kidney
Results from vascular interruption of the ureter at less than 15 weeks gestation.

Ovarian cyst
This is the most frequent cause of a cystic lower abdominal mass in the female fetus. The ovarian cysts may be 'simple' or theca lutein. The cysts may be unilocular or multiseptate. Large cysts up to 10 cm in diameter are occasionally seen.

Meconium pseudocyst
These develop in respect to the presence of meconium secondary to bowel perforation in utero. Perforation of the fetal bowel may be the result of bowel atresias/stenosis, volvulus, intussusception or cystic fibrosis, often resulting in peritoneal calcification.

Mesenteric cyst
Mesenteric cysts are thought to be lymphatic in origin and are reported to occur most commonly in the mesentery of the small bowel. Sonographically they usually have the appearances of a unilocular cystic mass but rarely a multiseptate appearance is seen.

Choledochal cyst
Usually seen in the subhepatic region, usually unilocular but may rarely have a multiseptate appearance. If the gallbladder is visible the cyst usually appears separate from it. Contiguous tubular cystic structures may suggest the diagnosis.

Retroperitoneal lymphangioma
Abdominal lymphangiomas most commonly involve the mesentery but are occasionally seen in the omentum or retroperitoneum. The majority of lymphangiomas are left sided. Lymphangiomas are usually multiloculate, although a unilocular cystic appearance has been described.

Hepatic mesenchymal hamartoma	Mesenchymal hamartomas of the liver usually present as a solitary round lesion with well defined margins consisting of multiple cysts of variable sizes separated by thick or thin septae.
Urachal cyst	Persistence of the urachal lumen without communication with the bladder or umbilicus may result in urachal cyst formation. These are seen as cystic structures adjacent to the dome of bladder behind the anterior abdominal wall.
Cystic teratoma	Teratomas may be ovarian or retroperitoneal and present a whole spectrum of US appearances. They may be solid, complex or cystic. If cystic they may be unilocular or multiseptate.
Torsion of ovarian cysts	The sonographic appearance of twisted ovarian cyst results in complex cystic masses that change with time.
Enteric duplication cyst	Enteric duplication cysts may occur at any point in the GIT. The stomach is less frequently affected than other regions. Duplication cysts are normally seen as thick-walled fluid collections, particularly if they do not communicate with the lumen of the bowel. They may occasionally be multiseptate.

Further Reading

Malnofski MJ, Poulton TB, Nazinithsy KJ & Hissong SL (1993) Prenatal ultrasonic diagnosis of retroperitoneal cystic lymphangioma. *J Ultrasound Med* 12: 427–429.

Nussabaum AR, Sanders RC, Hartman DS et al (1988) Neonatal ovarian cysts: sonographic–pathologic correlation. *Radiology* 1688: 817.

Ross PR, Olmsted WW, Moser RP Jr et al (1987) Mesenteric and omental cysts histologic classification with imaging correlation. *Radiology* 164: 327.

Shozu M, Akasof K, Yamashire G & Omura K (1993) Changing ultrasonographic appearances of fetal ovarian cyst twisted in utero. *J Ultrasound Med* 12: 415–417.

Solid Abdominal Masses in the Fetus

Normal bowel

This appears hyperechoic before 20 weeks.

Bowel masses

Causes include hyperechoic meconium (normal variant), meconium ileus, bowel obstruction with inspissated contents and meconium-filled rectum (a pseudomass). Cystic fibrosis should be considered. Echogenic bowel also described in trisomy 21 and IUGR.

Renal masses

Infantile (autosomal recessive) polycystic kidney disease, Wilms' tumor, dysplastic kidney, hamartoma, mesoblastic nephroma, ectopic kidney. Wilms' presents as a well-defined renal tumor with PH. PH is a consistent feature of renal tumors – decreased GIT uptake, compression by the mass and increased blood flow leading to increased urine production has been postulated as the cause of PH.

Normal adrenal gland

The fetal adrenal glands are relatively large in the third trimester and at birth are 20 times larger than in adult relative to body size. They are readily visualized in pregnancy as a bilaminar structure. The adrenal gland may be confused with a kidney in renal aplasia, particularly before 24 weeks.

Sacrococcygeal teratoma

These often protrude outwards from the fetal surface but intra-pelvic extension is common. They may be cystic or solid, the risk of malignancy being greater in solid lesions. Fetal and neonatal morbidity and mortality from SCT are in large part related to the vascularity of the tumor, which may act as a functional AV fistula with development of high output failure, hydrops and placentomegaly. Color flow Doppler/power Doppler may clearly demonstrate its extensive vascularity.

Hepatic masses	These include hepatoblastoma, hepatoma, hamartoma, hemangioma, metastases, hemangioendothelioma and hepatomegaly of any etiology.
Neuroblastoma	Neuroblastomas may occur anywhere along the sympathetic chain but the most common site is the adrenal gland. They may be solid or cystic.
Splenomegaly	Fetal splenomegaly is a common finding in rhesus isoimmunization and transplacental infections (see page 304).
Chordoma	Arising from remnants of the primitive notocord, these are rare tumors found in the sacrococcygeal and suboccipital regions of the spine, they are solid tumors.
Cystic mass with solid appearance	These are masses with internal hemorrhage or debris within them. Abdominal cystic hygroma can on rare occasions have a solid appearance on US.
Ovarian masses	Functional cysts are by far the most common ovarian masses in the fetus. Other ovarian masses which may occur in the ovary and may be solid are teratomas/dermoids.
Meningocele	Anterior meningocele is rare in the lower spine but may occur in the presacral region and is usually cystic. Solid elements within the cyst may represent glial tissue or lipoma.
Pulmonary sequestration	Extrathoracic pulmonary sequestration is reported to occur below the diaphragm. This has been reported in utero as a cause of solid upper abdominal masses.
Ectopic spleen	Ectopic spleen lying below the right kidney has been reported in a fetus with omphalocele.

Further Reading

Bousvaros A, Kirks DR & Grossman H (1986) Imaging of neuroblastoma: an overview. *Pediatr Radiol* 6: 89.

Comstock CH (1988) Fetal masses: ultrasound diagnosis and evaluation. *Ultrasound Q* 6: 229–236.

Ferraro EM, Fakhay T, Aruny JE et al (1989) Prenatal adrenal neuroblastoma: case report with review of the literature. *J Ultrasound Med* 7: 275–278.

Fowlie F, Giacomantonia M, McKenzie E et al (1986) Antenatal sonographic diagnosis of adrenal neuroblastoma. *J Can Assoc Radiol* 37: 50.

Fox DB, Bruner JP & Fleischer AC (1996) Amplitude-based color Doppler sonography of fetus with sacrococcygeal teratoma. *J Ultra Med* 15: 785–787.

Guilian BB, Chang CCN & Yass BS (1986) Prenatal ultrasonographic diagnosis of fetal adrenal neuroblastoma. *JCU* 14: 225.

Janetschek G, Weitzel D, Stein W et al (1986) Prenatal diagnosis of neuroblastoma by sonography. *Urology* 24: 397.

Paulson EK & Hetzberg BS (1991) Hyperechoic meconium in the third trimester fetus. *J Ultrasound Med* 10: 677–680.

Sohaey R, Woodward P & Zwiebel WJ (1996) Fetal G.I. anomalies. *Seminars in US, CT and MRI* 17(1): 51–65.

Suresh I, Suresh S, Arumuqum R et al (1997) Antenatal diagnosis of Wilms tumor. *J Ultra Med* 16: 69–72.

Dilated Loops of Fetal Bowel

Stomach

Pyloric atresia

Sonographic features include PH and dilatation of the stomach. The small bowel may be normally visualized because of the passage of bile.

Non-specific gastric dilatation

Transient non-specific dilatation of the stomach may present in normal fetuses. Repeat examination differentiates from pyloric atresia.

Small Bowel

Normal

The small bowel can be identified in the second trimester and normally measures 1.2 mm (range 1.0–1.5 mm) before 20 weeks gestation. The small bowel can be identified in only 30% of fetuses after 34 weeks.

Cystic fibrosis

Thirty-three per cent of fetuses presenting with dilated bowel distal to the duodenum have cystic fibrosis. Newborns presenting with large bowel obstruction have a 36% incidence of cystic fibrosis.

Meconium peritonitis

This is chemical peritonitis due to the presence of meconium released by a bowel perforation which may result in the formation of a pseudocyst or generalized ascites; fine particles within the ascites have been described as giving a 'snowstorm' appearance. Meconium deposits may calcify.

Small bowel atresia

Any segment of bowel may become atretic. The more distal the atresia, the lower the incidence of PH. Third trimester PH is only present in 20–30% of jejunal atresia.

Secondary to large bowel obstruction	Large bowel obstruction may occur as a result of anorectal atresia, Meconium plug syndrome, Hirschsprung's disease or megacystis-microcolon-intestinal hypoperistalsis syndrome (MMIHS).
Gastroschisis	Mild dilatation of the bowel is common with gastroschisis, and does not necessarily indicate obstruction, but marked dilatation may be secondary to bowel obstruction as a result of ischemia associated with volvulus. Bowel wall thickening is usually seen.
Midgut volvulus	Delayed return of the fetal midgut from the umbilical cord and failure of fixation results in malrotation. This may result in volvulus, bowel obstruction and ischemia of the small bowel.
Congenital chloridorrhea	A rare hereditary disorder characterized by impairment of active chloride transport from the distal ileum and colon. This results in dilated loops of bowel in utero. Associated PH has been reported.

Large Bowel

Hirschsprung's disease	The incidence of Hirschsprung's disease is 1:10 000. Dilated loops of bowel, PH and increase in abdominal circumference have been reported, although uncommon.
Meconium plug syndrome	Associated with cystic fibrosis.
Normal	Occasionally meconium in the fetus may appear echo-poor, mimicking dilated loops of bowel. The large bowel is easily visualized after 28 weeks. Large bowel lumen is seldom more than 1 cm in diameter at term.

Anorectal atresia	Imperforate anus occurs in approximately 1 in 5000 live births. More complex anorectal atresias are less common, and are frequently associated with fistulas into the urethra or perineum in males. Large bowel dilatation is occasionally evident on US. There may be features of associated sacral agenesis, lower limb hypoplasia or VACTERAL syndrome.
Megacystis microcolon (MMIHS)	Associated with functional small bowel obstruction, malrotation, microcolon and enlarged, non-obstructed urinary bladder. There may be associated hydronephrosis.

Further Reading

Anderson N, Malpas T & Robertson R (1995) Prenatal diagnosis of colon atresia. *Pediatr Radiol* 23: 63–65.

Babcook CJ, Hedrick MH, Goldstein RB et al (1994) Gastroschisis: can sonography accurately predict postnatal outcome? *J Ultrasound Med* 13: 701.

Estroff JA, Parod RB & Benacerraf BR (1992) Prevalence of cystic fibrosis in fetuses with dilated bowel. *Radiology* 183: 677–680.

Finley BE, Burlbaw J, Bennett TL & Levitch L (1992) Delayed return of the fetal midgut to the abdomen resulting in volvulus, bowel obstruction and gangrene of the small bowel. *J Ultrasound Med* 11: 233–235.

Goldstein I, Reec EA, Yarconic S et al (1987) Growth of the fetal stomach in normal pregnancies. *Obstet Gynecol* 70: 641.

Groli C, Zucca S & Cesarelli A (1986) Congenital chloridorrhea. Antenatal ultrasonic appearance. *JCU* 14: 253–259.

Haseqawa T, Kubota A, Imura K et al (1993) Prenatal diagnosis of congenital pyloric atresia. *JCU* 21: 278–281.

Hershkovitz E, Steiner Z, Shinwell ES et al (1994) Prenatal ultrasonic diagnosis of nonhypertrophic pyloric stenosis associated with malrotation. *JCU* 22(1): 52–54.

Hertzberg BS (1994) Sonography of the fetal gastrointestinal tract: anatomic variants, diagnostic pitfalls and abnormalities. *AJR* 162(5): 1175–1182.

Parulekar SG (1991) Sonography of normal fetal bowel. *J Ultrasound Med* 10: 211–220.

Satin AJ, Twickler DM & Wendal GD (1992) Congenital syphilis associated with dilatation of fetal small bowel. *J Ultrasound Med* 11: 49–52.

Stamm E, King G & Thickman D (1991) Megacystis microcolon-intestinal hypoperistalsis syndrome: prenatal identification in siblings and review of the literature. *J Ultrasound Med* 10: 599–602.

Vermesh M, Mayden KL, Canfino E et al (1986) Prenatal sonographic diagnosis of Hirschsprung's disease. *J Ultrasound Med* 5: 27–34.

Increased Echogenicity in Fetal Abdomen

Intra-abdominal calcification	Scattered foci of increased echogenicity in the distribution of the liver, spleen and peritoneal cavity, with or without acoustic shadowing, usually secondary to in utero perforation.
Meconium peritonitis	This is the most common cause of abdominal calcification, it may be associated with dilated loops of bowel and PH. Cystic fibrosis should be considered.
Meconium pseudocyst	A cystic mass with hyperechoic margins secondary to perforation.
Transplacental infections	Toxoplasmosis, CMV, varicella cause liver calcification.
Portal vein thrombosis	Portal vein thrombosis may show calcification in the portal vein distribution but portal vein thromboemboli may resemble other causes of hepatic calcifications, i.e. infections.
Atretic bowel segment	Intramural calcification may occur in an atretic bowel segment.
Neoplasia	Many abdominal neoplasms, including neuroblastoma, teratoma, hemangioma and hepatoblastoma, are known to calcify in neonates.
Calcified IVC and renal vein thrombus	Uncommon. Combined thrombosis of IVC and renal vein is an uncommon occurrence in the neonate and is extremely rare in utero. Hyperechoic streaks in the distribution of the IVC and renal vein are noted and may shadow. Venous collaterals may be demonstrated by Doppler.
Urinary ascites	A rare cause of peritoneal calcification in the neonate following bladder or pelvicalyceal rupture secondary to obstruction.

Tissue necrosis	Tissue necrosis is a well known cause of calcification. Ischemic hepatic necrosis as a cause of fetal hepatic calcification has been reported.
Hyperdense intramural material	Dense structures such as inspissated meconium/ meconium ileus and hematomas often cause increased fetal abdominal echogenicity, usually in obstructed bowel.
Multiple interfaces	Rhabdomyosarcomas are exceedingly rare tumors that may occur in a neonate. They have multiple reflective interfaces.
Air within the fetus	This is usually secondary to fetal demise. An echo pattern consistent with gas in the large bowel of a live fetus has been reported, presumably secondary to amnionitis.
Fat	Lipomas, if detected prenatally, may conceivably cause increased echogenicity.
Normal variant	In early to midpregnancy hyperdense bowel is normal.

Further Reading

Capsi B, Elchalal U, Hagay Z et al (1993) Echogenicity of fetal bowel due to gas accumulation. *J Ultrasound Med* 4: 231-233.

Fung ASL, Wilson S, Toi A & Johnson JA (1992) Echogenic colonic meconium in the third trimester: a normal sonographic finding. *J Ultrasound Med* 11: 676-678.

Lalmand B, Avni EF, Nasr A et al (1990) Prenatal renal vein thrombosis: sonographic demonstration. *J Ultrasound Med* 9: 437.

Lince DM, Pretorius DH, Manco-Johnson ML et al (1985) The clinical significance of increased echogenicity in the fetal abdomen. *AJR* 145: 683-686.

Nguyan DL & Leonard JC (1986) Ischemic hepatic necrosis. A cause of fetal liver calcification. *AJR* L467: 596-597.

Parulekar SG (1991) Sonography of normal fetal bowel. *J Ultrasound Med* 10: 211-220.

Paulson EK & Hertzberg BS (1992) Hyperechoic meconium in the third trimester. A normal sonographic finding. *J Ultrasound Med* 11: 676-678.

Radner M, Vergesslich KA & Weninger M (1993) Meconium peritonitis: a new finding in rubella syndrome. *JCU* 21: 346-349.

Rypens F, Avni F, Braude P et al (1993) Calcified inferior vena cava thrombus in a fetus: prenatal imaging. *J Ultrasound Med* 12: 55–58.

Rypens F, Avni F, Abehsera MM et al (1995) Areas of increased echogenicity in the fetal abdomen; diagnosis and significance. *Radiographics* 15: 1329–1331.

Stein B, Bromley B, Michlewitz H et al (1995) Fetal liver calcifications: sonographic appearance and postnatal outcome. *Radiology* 197(2): 489–492.

Weiner Z (1995) Congenital cytomegalovirus infections with oligohydramnios and echogenic bowel at 14 weeks gestation. *J Ultrasound Med* 14: 617–618.

Causes of Fetal Ascites

Hydrops fetalis
Fetal ascites may occur as a part of hydrops.

Hematologic
The hematologic causes of fetal ascites include: Rh isoimmunization, fetal hemoglobinopathy, 6GPD deficiency, fetal hemorrhage, twin–twin transfusion and anemia due to maternal-acquired pure red cell aplasia.

Infections
Transplacental infections that have been associated with fetal ascites include coxsackie, CMV, parvo-virus, RSV, herpes simplex type I, toxoplasmosis and syphilis.

Gastrointestinal
Causes include bowel atresias, volvulus, meconium peritonitis and bowel obstruction with perforation.

Genitourinary
Urinary tract obstructions with perforation.

Metabolic
Storage diseases and other metabolic disorders, e.g. Gaucher's disease, mucopolysaccharidosis.

Hepatobiliary
Congenital hepatic tumors, hepatitis in utero and biliary atresia.

Abdominal neoplasia
Mostly intra-abdominal tumors but extra-abdominal tumors such as neuroblastoma and teratoma have also been associated with ascites.

Respiratory
Ascites may complicate any major pulmonary abnormality, including congenital cystic adenomatoid malformation, pulmonary lymphangiectasia, congenital tumors, extralobar sequestration, chylothorax, diaphragmatic hernia or enlargement of one lung, by obstructing venous return to the right atrium.

Pseudoascites

This represents an artifact and is seen as a linear lucency beneath the skin on the lateral part of the abdomen. This artifact is said to relate to the cone-like shape of the fetal abdomen with a contribution from the muscles of the abdominal wall.

Further Reading

Adzick NS, Harrison MR, Flake AW et al (1985) Urinary extravasation in the fetus with obstructive uropathy. *J Pediatr Surg* 20: 608.

Hasimoto BE, Filly RA, Callan PW (1986) Fetal pseudo ascites: further anatomic observations. *J Ultrasound Med* 5: 151.

Sanders RC (1986) *Atlas of Ultrasonographic Artifact and Variants*, p. 15. Chicago Year Book Medical.

Causes of Fetal Hepatomegaly

Transplacental infection	These include viral infections such as CMV, rubella, coxsackie and varicella. Other associated infections include toxoplasmosis and syphilis.
Hemolysis	Rh incompatibility, isoimmunization and congenital hemolytic anemia, e.g. spherocytosis.
Venous congestion	Congenital heart disease with right-sided and biventricular heart failure.
Hepatic masses	These are mostly neoplastic and include hemangioma, mesenchymal hamartoma, hepatoblastoma, hepatic adenoma, hemangiopericytoma and metastases, e.g. neuroblastoma. Solitary cysts or polycystic disease of the liver may also cause hepatomegaly.
Metabolic	These include galactosemia, trypsinemia, α-1 antitrypsin deficiency, disorders of the urea cycle, methylmalonic acidemia and sialidosis.
Beckwith–Wiedemann syndrome	Sonographic features include visceromegaly, hemihypertrophy, increased renal cortical echogenicity, omphalocele or umbilical hernia.
Zellweger's syndrome	Sonography may reveal limb anomalies such as talipes equinovarus, rocker-bottom feet, bell-shaped thorax, cerebral ventricular dilatation and renal cysts. Analysis of amniotic fluid reveals deficiency of the enzyme dihydroxyacetone phosphate acyltransferase in the amniotic fluid cells, and the absence of peroxisomes in cultured amniotic fluid cells.

Further Reading

Romero R, Pilu G, Jeanty P et al (1989) *Prenatal Diagnosis of Congenital Anomalies*, p. 250. Norwalk, CT: Appleton & Lange.

Fetal Liver Masses

Hepatic cyst	Hepatic cysts are not uncommon.
Choledochal cyst	These cysts vary in size and location within the liver or juxtaposition to the liver. The cyst appears in the expected location of the bile ducts. Tubular structures are seen entering the cyst.
Mesenchymal hepatic hamartoma	Usually present as solitary round lesions with well-defined margins consisting of multiple cysts of variable sizes, separated by thick or thin septa. Antenatal detection has been reported at 25 weeks.
Hemangioma	These may be solid, cystic or complex. Cavernous hemangiomas are the most common: high output failure, hydrops and intrauterine death have been reported. Doppler US may demonstrate increased flow within these masses, and help differentiate cystic tumors from other cystic masses.
Hepatic teratoma	In common with teratomas elsewhere these may vary from solid to completely cystic masses, although most tumors are complex.
Portal vein aneurysm	This is usually seen as a focal dilatation of the portal vein; color flow Doppler/pulsed Doppler sonography demonstrates active blood flow within the mass.
Hepatoblastoma	Usually a solid tumor.
Hepatic adenoma	Very rare in the newborn but have been reported in utero. Adenomas are seen as hypoechoic masses with irregular margins. Adenomas reported in utero may be associated with maternal treatment with steroids and other hormones during pregnancy.

Hepatic
hemangioendothelioma

Benign, highly vascular, usually diagnosed in
infancy. Benign but life-threatening condition
that may cause high output failure from AV
shunting, consumptive coagulopathy and liver
rupture usually associated with raised alpha
fetoprotein and cutaneous hemangioma. US:
hepatomegaly, heterogeneous solid, cystic (uni-
locular/multilocular) or complex mass, hyperechoic, hypoechoic or mixed echogenicity.
There is increased fetal abdominal circumference. The maternal αFP was elevated in one
case but was associated with placental chorioangioma. Non-immune hydrops due to CCF may
ensue. The AV shunting within the tumor may
be demonstrated with color Doppler.

Fetal Liver Calcifications

Ischemic/vascular accident	Ischemic hepatic necrosis with secondary vascular thrombosis following anemic shock from an in utero placental accident. Portal vein thrombosis (? Embolization of liver from thrombosis in central veins).

Infections

- CMV
- TORCH (Toxoplasmosis, rubella, CMV, Herpes simplex)
- Meconium peritonitis (chemical)

Neoplasia

- Hemangioma
- Hamartoma (benign)
- Hepatocellular carcinoma
- Hepatoblastoma (malignant)

Gallstones in a contracted GB	When GB is contracted echogenic foci within the GB may not be perceived as gallstones and misdiagnosed as liver or peritoneal calcification. Further imaging with this possibility in mind may demonstrate a crescent of bile/gallbladder.

Idiopathic

Further Reading

Abuhamad AZ, Lewis D, Inati MN et al (1993) The use of color flow Doppler in the diagnosis of fetal hepatic hemangioma. *J Ultrasound Med* 4: 223–226.

Chuileanain FN, Rowlands S, Sampion (1999) Ultrasonographic appearances of fetal hepatic hemangioma. *J Ultra Med* 18: 379–381.

Eirad H, Mayden KL, Ahowt S et al (1985) Prenatal ultrasound diagnosis of choledochal cyst. *J Ultrasound Med* 4: 553–556.

Hertzberg BS & Kliewer MA (1998) Fetal gallstones in a contracted gallbladder: potential to simulate hepatic or peritoneal calcification. *J Ultra Med* 17: 667–670.

Marks F, Thomas P, Lustig I et al (1990) In utero sonographic description of a fetal liver adenoma. *J Ultrasound Med* 8: 112–119.

Meirowitz NB, Guzman ER, Underberg-Davis SJ et al (2000) Hepatic hemangio-endothelioma: Prenatal sonographic findings and evaluation of the lesion. *JCU* 28: 258–263.

Richards DS, Cruz AC, Dowdy KA (1988) Prenatal diagnosis of fetal liver calcifications. *J Ultra Med* 7: 691–694.

Stein B, Bromley B, Michlewitz H et al (1995) Fetal liver calcifications: sonographic appearance and outcome. *Radiology* 197: 489–492.

Echogenic Material Within the Fetal Gallbladder

Sludge
: The echogenicity of gallbladder sludge varies from highly reflective to subtle sludge layers and does not shadow. Difficulty may arise occasionally in differentiating tiny calculi from sludge.

Gallstones
: Have been seen antenatally. They may resolve spontaneously after birth.

Non-Visualization of Fetal Gallbladder

The gallbladder can be seen in most fetuses (82.5%) in the second and the third trimester. The significance of non-visualization of a gallbladder as a sign of fetal abnormality is therefore uncertain, but the sign may be significant when scanning fetuses, whose parents are both carriers of cystic fibrosis. Most fetuses with non-visualization have a normal outcome. Causes of fetal non-visualization of gallbladder:

- Normal fetuses (5%)
- Cystic fibrosis
- Biliary atresia
- Gallbladder atresia
- Trisomy 21 (coincidental ? single case reported)

Further Reading

Chan L, Rao BK, Jiang Y et al (1995) Fetal gallbladder growth and development during gestation. *J Ultra Med* 14: 421–423.

Devonald KJ, Ellwood DA & Colditz PB (1992) The variable appearances of fetal gallstones. *J Ultrasound Med* 11: 579–585.

Hertzberg BS, Kliewer MA, Maynor C et al (1996) Non-visualisation of the gallbladder: frequency and prognostic importance. *Radiology* 199: 679–682.

Suchet IB, Labafle MF, Dycke CS et al (1993) Fetal cholelithiasis. A case report and review of the literature. *J Clin Ultrasound* 21: 198–202.

Causes of Fetal Splenomegaly

Transplacental infections	These include viral infections such as CMV, rubella, coxsackie and infections with toxoplasma and syphilis.
Hematologic disorders	These include Rh incompatibility, hemolytic and other anemias, often associated with FH.
Congestive cardiac failure	This may be associated with major cardiac defects, cardiomegaly or arrythmias.
Metabolic disorders/ storage diseases	Gaucher's disease, Niemann–Pick disease, Wolman's disease, hypothyroidism and galactosemia.
Beckwith–Wiedemann syndrome	Associated with visceromegaly and skeletal anomalies.
Space-occupying lesions of spleen	Splenomegaly has been identified with splenic cysts and hamartomas.
Congenital neoplasia/ malignancy	Splenomegaly has been reported in association with congenital leukemia, lymphoma and histiocytosis.

NB The spleen can be identified in most fetuses between 18 and 40 weeks. In the fetus the spleen is of similar echogenicity as the kidney. Ectopic spleen lying below the right kidney has been reported in a fetus with omphalocele.

Fetal Splenic Aplasia/Hypoplasia

Hypoplastic spleen

The spleen is not clearly visualized; splenic hypoplasia may be associated with Di George's syndrome and sickle cell anemia.

Splenic aplasia

True splenic aplasia is rare and may be hereditary or secondary to exposure to warfarin in utero.

Further Reading

Schmidt W, Yarkoni S, Jeanty P et al (1985) Sonographic measurements of fetal spleen: clinical implications. *J Ultrasound Med* 4: 667.

8

Fetal Genitourinary System

Fetal Renal Biometry

The fetal kidneys initially appear as hypoechogenic regions. As pregnancy advances, there is deposition of fat in the perinephric region, and differentiation of cortex from medulla is apparent in most fetuses by 24 weeks. Amniotic fluid volume assessment is vital. The fetal bladder can be visualized in all normal fetuses. (The bladder may be empty immediately postmicturition. If the bladder is not seen rescan after an interval.)

Normal kidney function
: Kidneys produce urine from the 10th week gestation, by the 15th week urine forms a major component of AF. Early in the second term, the fetal kidneys are isoechoic to the adjacent viscera. The kidney length should normally measure approximately 1 mm for each week of gestation through the second and third trimester. With advancing pregnancy and with laying down of retroperitoneal fat and renal collecting system fat the kidneys become much more well-defined ultrasonically.

Assessment of urine production
: Serial volume measurements of the fetal bladder can give a rough assessment of urine production. Bladder volume = bladder dimensions AP × transverse × length × 0.52 (ml). The fetal bladder normally empties every 30–45 minutes.

Fetal diuretic stress test

Diuresis induced in the mother by the administration of a powerful diuretic is said to help clarify cases of severe OH late in pregnancy. Diuresis may cause a significant increase in urine output in the fetus but failure of diuretic effect in a compromised pregnancy may be the result of poor renal perfusion rather than a result of renal agenesis or dysplasia. The utility of this test may be limited and clinical judgment is made in each case specifically. As is often the case in OH, visualization of fetal parts is limited, differentiation between chronic fetal compromise and renal output failure may therefore be difficult.

Further Reading

Hammond DI (1992) Prenatal diagnosis of urinary tract malformations. *J Can Assoc Radiol* 43(3): 179-187.

Sanders RC (1992) In utero sonography of genitourinary anomalies. *Urol Radiol* 43(3): 29-33.

Seeds JW (1998) Borderline genitourinary tract abnormalities. *Seminars Ultrasound, CT & MRI* 19: 347-354.

Zhou Q, Cardoza JD, Barth R (1999) Prenatal sonography of congenital renal malformations. *AJR* 173: 1371-1376.

Empty Fetal Renal Fossa

Pelvic kidney

When one renal fossa is empty, a search for the kidneys in ectopic positions should be made. If the contralateral kidney is of normal size the obvious place to search for a kidney is the pelvis. Ectopic kidneys may be associated with other urinary tract anomalies.

Renal agenesis

During the 5th week of gestation, the ureteral buds arise. If the ureteral buds do not develop renal agenesis occurs. Severe OH develops with bilateral renal agenesis resulting in pulmonary hypoplasia (Potter's syndrome). The diagnosis of pulmonary hypoplasia may not be reliably made on antenatal US. Bilateral renal agenesis is relatively common: 1:3000–4000.

Hypoplastic kidney

Renal hypoplasia may be unilateral or bilateral and the small kidney may be difficult to locate. The contralateral kidney may be hypertrophied but if it is also small then there may be OH. Renal hypoplasia may also be associated with other anomalies.

Crossed renal ectopia

A kidney with a bilobed contour, with two areas of increased echogenicity representing the collecting systems, is seen in one renal fossa. A kidney in the contralateral renal fossa would not be seen. As expected the crossed ectopic kidney will be longer than a normal kidney.

Horse-shoe kidney

The kidney is more inferiorly placed and therefore the renal fossa may appear empty. This is the most common renal fusion anomaly with two distinct renal units lying on either side of the midline but connected at their lower poles by a renal parenchymal or fibrous isthmus crossing the midline. May be an isolated anomaly or occur with other renal anomalies. 30% associated with other anomalies: skeletal, CVS, CNS and anorectal malformations. 25% are associated with other genitourinary abnormalities: duplication, ureterocele uretero-vesical reflux, undescended testis, hypospadius, bicornuate uterus or septate vagina. There is also an association with trisomy 21 (20%), trisomy 18 and Turners syndrome (60%). US diagnosis is achieved by multiple transverse and coronal scans at different levels between the upper and lower poles of both kidneys. Post-natal follow up is important because of the high likelihood of malrotation and obstruction of the ureters.

NB A prominent adrenal gland or bowel loop in the renal fossa may mimic the kidney, making diagnosis difficult. The normal fetal kidney after 22 weeks gestation will show corticomedullary differentiation.

Further Reading

Collay N & Hooker JG (1989) Prenatal diagnosis of pelvic kidney. *Prenatal Diagn* 9: 361.

Kovo-Hasharoni M, Mashiach R, Levi S and Meizner I (1997) Prenatal sonographic diagnosis of horse-shoe kidney. *JCU* 25: 405–407.

MacKenzie FM, Kingston GO & Oppenheimer L (1994) Early prenatal diagnosis of bilateral renal agenesis using transvaginal sonography and color Doppler ultrasonography. *J Ultrasound Med* 13: 49–51.

Meizner I & Barnhard Y (1995) Bilateral fetal pelvic kidneys documentation of two cases of a rare prenatal finding. *J Ultrasound Med* 14: 487.

Meizner I, Yitzhak A, Levi A et al (1995) Fetal pelvic kidney: a challenge in prenatal diagnosis? *Ultrasound Obstetrics & Gynecology* 5: 391.

Sherer DM, Jacquelyn BH, Cullen MD et al (1990) Prenatal sonographic findings associated with a fetal horse shoe kidney. *J Ultrasound Med* 9: 477–479.

Enlarged Fetal Kidneys

Hydronephrosis

Hydronephrosis is the most common cause of a neonatal abdominal mass and often results from PUJ obstruction. Other causes of hydronephrosis include VUJ obstruction, vesicoureteric reflux, bladder outlet obstruction/urethral valves, etc. Antenatally, hydronephrosis is usually readily identified, however, gross hydronephrosis may be confused with multicystic dysplastic kidney.

Multicystic dysplastic kidney

MDK represent a mass of disorganized tissue including cartilage, cysts and abnormal tubules which develop when the distal ureteric bud is atretic resulting in a multicystic dysplastic kidney (Potters type 2). An MDK is non-functioning and when bilateral results in OH and lethal pulmonary hypoplasia. The majority of cases are unilateral; when bilateral the condition is fatal. US features depend upon the subtype. In pattern type IIa the kidney is seen as a large paraspinal flank mass. It contains cysts of various sizes, separated by solid tissue. In type IIb multiple renal cysts are associated with renal pelvic dilatation. Type IIa is the most common. It is thought to be due to interruption to the vascular supply to the ureter resulting in ureteric atresia before 15 weeks gestation. US: echogenic mass with cortical cysts of varying size randomly distributed.

Infantile polycystic kidney disease (IPKD)

Autosomal recessive polycystic kidney; the kidneys are enlarged and echogenic due to the presence of multiple small cysts. The cysts are too small to be resolved sonographically. IPKD may be associated with OH and hepatic fibrosis.

Cystic renal dysplasia
with obstruction
(Potters type 4)

In this abnormality the kidneys develop normally initially but then with increasing outflow obstruction; early on in pregnancy hydronephrosis and renal dysplasia develop. The renal collecting system may rupture giving rise to a perinephric urinoma. The condition is usually bilateral and more common in male fetuses. It occurs most commonly in fetuses with distended bladder and posterior urethral valves. OH may lead to poor prognosis. US features are variable, the kidneys are abnormally echogenic. There are renal cortical cysts of varying sizes associated with hydronephrosis. In fetal kidneys with evidence of urinary tract obstruction, sonographic demonstration of cortical cysts effectively indicates the presence of cystic renal dysplasia. However, the absence of visible cysts does not exclude cystic dysplasia. The kidneys may not usually be enlarged.

Mesoblastic nephroma

Usually unilateral. Sonographically mesoblastic nephroma is seen as a large, solitary, predominantly solid, coarse, echogenic renal mass which may contain cystic areas. It may be associated with PH.

Heredofamilial cystic
dysplasia

Cystic renal dysplasia is an important feature of several familial syndromes. The Meckel–Gruber syndrome is a recessive inherited condition associated with bilateral non-obstructive multicystic dysplastic kidneys, occipital encephalocele and postaxial polydactyly. Other syndromes associated with non-obstructive renal dysplasia include:
(1)   Asphyxiating thoracic dystrophy
(2)   Short rib-polydactyly syndrome
(3)   Trisomy 13
(4)   Holoprosencephaly.

Nephroblastomatosis	Nephroblastomatosis is the persistence of primitive blastema in an abnormal location and/or abnormal quantity. US reveals bilateral nephromegaly with normal renal echogenicity, but foci or calcification may be associated with PH and can occur as a part of a familial condition – Perlman's syndrome, which includes nephroblastomatosis, fetal ascites, macrosomia and Wilms' tumor.
Adult type polycystic disease (Potters type 3)	Autosomal dominant; the condition usually presents in adults but has been diagnosed in the fetus. The kidneys may be enlarged as a result of cystic dilatation of the tubules and glomeruli, associated with increased echogenicity mimicking autosomal recessive disease but sometimes the cortical renal cysts may be sufficiently large to be visible on US, which can confirm the diagnosis when it occurs in the fetus of a parent with the disease. As there is adequate renal function in utero there is no OH.
Beckwith–Wiedemann syndrome	This syndrome may be associated with omphalocele (12% of cases) and organomegaly. There is an increased incidence of hemi-hypertrophy, renal anomalies, Wilms' tumor and hepatoblastoma.
Metabolic disorders	Tyrosinemia type I is inherited in an autosomal recessive manner. Symptoms may present acutely or adopt a more chronic form. Presentation is usually in infancy. Sonographic manifestations include nephromegaly and features of cirrhosis. Prenatal diagnosis may be achieved by amniocentesis or chorionic villous sampling. Glycogen storage disease type I and type IIa may both present in infancy; nephromegaly is a common feature.

| Asphyxiating thoracic dystrophy | This short-limbed osteochondrodysplasia occurs almost exclusively in Caucasians. The sonographic features include renal cysts, a narrow thorax, with or without rhizomelic shortening and with or without polydactyly. |
| Renal vein thrombosis | See page 316. |

Further Reading

Ambrosino MM, Heranz-Schulman M, Horii SC et al (1990) Prenatal diagnosis of nephroblastomatosis in live siblings. *J Ultrasound Med* 9: 49–51.

Geirsson RT, Ricketts NEM, Taylor DJ et al (1985) Prenatal appearance of mesoblastic nephroma associated with polyhydramnios. *JCU* 12: 488.

Gloor JM, Ogburn PL Jr, Beckle RJ et al (1995) Urinary tract anomalies detected by prenatal ultrasound examination at Mayo Clinic Rochester. *Radiology* 197: 559 (abstract).

Kvittinger EA, Guibaud PP, Divry P et al (1986) Prenatal diagnosis of hereditary/tyrosinaemia type I by determination of fumarylacetoacetate in chorionic villus material. *Eur J Pediatr* 144: 597.

Zhou Q, Cardoza JD & Barth R (1999) Prenatal sonography of congenital renal malformations. *AJR* 173: 1371–1376.

Cystic Fetal Kidneys

Obstructed kidneys

Obstructed kidneys or an obstructed upper moiety of a duplex system may mimic renal cysts; with careful attention to detail no confusion should normally arise.

Infantile polycystic disease

In this autosomal recessive polycystic kidney disease, large echogenic kidneys are seen. The cysts are usually too small to be resolved sonographically; however very small cysts are occasionally visible with modern scanners.

Adult-type polycystic disease

This autosomal dominant disease has now been reported in the fetus, newborns and juveniles as well as adults. Sonography reveals increased echogenicity in enlarged kidneys (85%) and renal cysts of varying sizes (58%). Cysts can be visualized in utero in some cases.

Multicystic dysplastic kidneys

These are common and are seen as enlarged cystic kidneys. These kidneys do not function. If bilateral, it is a lethal abnormality.

Cystic renal dysplasia

Caused by obstruction to urinary drainage, most frequently of the urethra but also at the level of the PUJ. In fetal kidneys with evidence of urinary tract obstruction US demonstration of cortical cysts effectively indicates the presence of cystic renal dysplasia as early as 21 weeks gestation. However, the absence of visible cysts does not exclude cystic dysplasia.

Cystic renal tumors

Mesoblastic nephroma is the most common congenital renal neoplasm. It is a solitary hamartoma, usually benign. Sonographically mesoblastic nephroma is seen as a complex mass which may contain cystic areas. It may be associated with PH. Wilms' tumor may also present as a multiloculated mass.

Heredofamilial cystic dysplasia

Cystic renal dysplasia is an important feature of several familial syndromes. Renal cysts have been described in association with over 50 syndromes. These include the trisomies, von Hippel-Lindau disease, Jeune's asphyxiating thoracic dystrophy, Meckel–Gruber syndrome, short rib-polydactyly syndrome, Beckwith–Wiedemann syndrome and holoprosencephaly.

Medullary cyst disease

This condition is characterized by cysts within the renal medulla which may result in tubular atrophy and subsequent renal failure. It usually manifests itself in the adult but is rarely seen in the newborn, with similar pathological findings.

Further Reading

Narain K, Pretorius DH, Reznik UM et al (1993) Spectrum of clinical presentation in fetal cystic renal disease: case report. *J Ultrasound Med* 112: 757-760.

Pretorius DH, Lee MH, Manco-Johnson ML et al (1987) Diagnoses of autosomal dominant polycystic kidney disease in utero and in the young infant. *J Ultrasound Med* 6: 249-255.

Echogenic Fetal Kidneys

Infantile renal polycystic disease (Potters Type 1)

Autosomal recessive; causing cystic dilatation of collecting tubules. The cystic dilatation does not result in macroscopic cysts but gives rise to multiple interfaces giving rise to enlarged bilateral echogenic kidneys. If renal function is poor OH may develop. There is an association with hepatic fibrosis. If the infant survives early childhood hepatic fibrosis may lead to death from hepatic failure and portal hypertension.

Adult polycystic disease (Potters Type 3)

See page 312.

Cystic renal dysplasia with obstruction (Potters Type 4)

Cysts associated with hydronephrosis usually due to urethral obstruction and OH (see page 311).

Renal vein thrombosis

Large hyperechoic kidney or voluminous echogenic mass in the third trimester. Initially the kidney is enlarged and hyperechoic, as enlargement is progressive asymmetry becomes obvious; if concomitant adrenal hematoma is present it contributes to the asymmetry. Hyperechoic streaks in a vascular pattern in the interlobular spaces and/or around the pyramids converging towards the hilum may be evident. Color Doppler confirms the absence of flow in the renal vein thrombosis and is associated with an increased pulsatility index in the ipsilateral kidney. At a later stage if resolution occurs there is a reduction in renal size with reappearance of venous flow in a recannulated vein or via collateral veins. With progressive disease calcification may appear within the thrombosed vein and the kidney; renal atrophy finally occurs. The kidneys may be enlarged with loss of corticomedullary differentiation in the neonate. There is an increased incidence in diabetes.

Trisomy 13	The combination of holoprosencephaly, facial clefting, CHD, polydactyly, dysplastic large echogenic kidneys suggest the diagnosis of trisomy 13.
Beckwith–Wiedemann syndrome	Large echogenic kidneys associated with macrosomia, hepatomegaly, splenomegaly, macroglossia and omphalocele suggest the diagnosis.
Meckel–Gruber syndrome	Large echogenic kidneys occasionally associated with cortical cysts and polydactyly and encephalocele.
Cytomegalovirus infection	Large echogenic kidneys with normal urinary bladder and mild/moderate PH have been described with CMV infections. No other fetal abnormality was recorded, although postnatal sonography demonstrated mild hydrocephalus and echogenic foci in the basal ganglia and thalami, suggestive of a transplacental infection.
Normal variant with normal AF	In hyperechoic kidneys with normal AF, a poor prognosis cannot be assumed.
Congenital Finnish nephrosis	This is a protein-losing nephropathy due to congenital abnormality of the glomeruli. There is a marked increase in α-fetoprotein both in amniotic fluid and maternal serum as a result of protein leakage into fetal urine. The kidneys are hyperechoic but may appear of normal size and echogenic.

Further Reading

Choong KKL, Gruenewald SM & Hodson EM (1993) Echogenic fetal kidneys in cytomegalovirus infections. *JCU* 21: 128–132.

Fishman JE & Joseph RC (1994) Renal vein thrombosis in utero: duplex sonography in diagnosis and follow up. *Pediatr Radiol* 24(2): 135–136.

Lalmand B, Avni EF, Nasr A et al (1990) Perinatal renal vein thrombosis. Sonographic demonstration. *J Ultrasound Med* 9: 437.

Anquenot J-L (1999) Antenatal renal vein thrombosis after accidental electric shock in a pregnant woman. *J Ultrasound Med* 18: 779–881.

Fetal Urinary Tract Dilatation

PUJ obstruction

Hydronephrosis is the most common cause of a neonatal abdominal mass and often results from PUJ obstruction. Approximately 10–30% of PUJ obstructions are bilateral, but involvement is usually asymmetric and severe bilateral obstruction is rare. In rare cases the renal pelvis may dilate to create a giant abdominal cyst with little or no recognizable renal parenchyma. OH may result with severe bilateral obstruction and, paradoxically, PH may also occur in 25% of cases. A urinoma or urinary ascites may result from urinary tract rupture in utero. A PUJ obstruction may be suspected when there is marked hydronephrosis with a prominent renal pelvis without hydroureter. Identical appearances may occur with severe vesicoureteric reflux if the ureter is not distended with urine at the time of scanning.

Vesicoureteric reflux

Vesicoureteric reflux is suspected by the presence of dilatation of the renal tract that varies with time. Intermittent dilatation of the ureter is a strong indicator of reflux.

Vesicoureteric junction obstruction

VUJ obstruction may occur in isolation or in association with a duplex kidney and double ureters. In duplex kidneys, the ureter from the upper renal moiety inserts into the bladder or distal urinary tract at a low ectopic site. This ectopic ureter is prone to obstruct and may dilate and herniate into the bladder or urethra as a ureterocele. The upper moiety may thus become hydronephrotic: a dilated ureter from obstruction is seen as a cystic serpiginous tubular structure in the lower abdomen running behind the bladder. Dilatation of the lower moiety is likely to be due to reflux.

Multicystic dysplastic
kidney type IIb

In type IIb disease there are multiple cysts of varying sizes accompanied by dilatation of the renal pelvis. The multicystic dysplastic kidney has no significant function.

Urethral obstruction

Urethral obstruction occurs more frequently in males than females and is most commonly due to posterior urethral valves. Obstruction to bladder emptying results in persistent dilatation of the bladder, thickened bladder wall and dilated collecting systems. Urinary ascites, urinomas and dystrophic bladder wall calcification are often associated abnormalities which may occur. Oligohydramnios indicates a poor prognosis. It may be associated with cystic dysplastic changes in the renal parenchyma. Dilated bladder is seen in the female in cloacal abnormalities.

Duplex systems

Duplex kidney may be difficult to diagnose antenatally unless hydronephrosis is present. However there may be certain pointers to the diagnosis, which include a larger kidney on the affected side and with careful scanning two renal collecting systems may be demonstrated. Hydronephrosis in one duplex system moiety is usually associated with a ureterocele. Sonography may show a dilated ureter on the affected side in association with a ureterocele which can often be demonstrated within the bladder. An ectopic ureter should be suspected with upper moiety hydronephrosis.

Miscellaneous non-obstructive dilatations	Generalized or focal non-obstructive dilatation may be seen in infants in congenital mega-calyces, exomphalos, macroglossia, Beckwith–Wiedemann syndrome and the Laurence–Moon–Biedl syndrome. Rarely, dilated calyces may be seen in ectopic, malrotated fused kidneys. In primary megaureter, dilatation is usually confined to the ureters only. Chromosomal abnormalities have been reported in association with PUJ obstruction, bladder outlet obstruction and mild pelvic dilatation, but this is uncommon.
Prune belly syndrome	The syndrome is characterized by severe deficiency of abdominal wall musculature associated with gross dilatation of the bladder and ureters. The collecting system dilatation is non-obstructive. Despite the presence of gross ureteric dilatation the kidneys are small and the calyces may not be particularly dilated. It may result from resolution of urinary ascites in utero.
Megacystis-microcolon intestinal hypoperistalsis syndrome	The syndrome comprises of small bowel obstruction, microcolon and megacystis. US: dilated bladder associated with bilateral hydro-nephrosis and a dilated fluid-filled stomach.
Pressure from pelvic masses	Ovarian masses, anterior meningocele, pelvic sacrococcygeal teratoma and hydrocolpos may compress the urinary bladder and/or the lower ureters, causing upper renal tract dilatation.

Pyelectasis and neonatal intervention

Normally the fetal renal pelvis is either not seen or visualized as a tiny streak of fluid collection placed on the medial aspect of the kidney. As to whether neonatal intervention would be required for renal pelvic dilatation is based on AP measurement of the renal pelvis. In general the greater the AP diameter of the renal pelvis, the greater the likelihood of neonatal intervention. Progressive dilatation or associated caliectasis greatly increase the probability of neonatal renal intervention. Normal AP diameter = <5 mm, usually there are no cases of intervention <9 mm, no intervention is required <5 mm up to 20 weeks gestation and <7 mm in up to 33 weeks gestation. An isolated pyelactasis is less likely to lead to intervention but intervention is more likely in association with caliectasis.

Mild pyelectasis and aneuploidy

Few if any fetuses with mild pyelectasis 4–5 mm at less than 20 weeks gestation are associated with significant fetal pathology. Mild pyelectasis 4 mm or greater is associated with trisomy 21 (25%).

Recurrence of mild familial pyelectasis

Recurrence of mild pyelectasis within families has been described, which appear to be linked to a single gene disorder and is not associated with renal dysfunction.

NB After 19 weeks gestation measurement of the AP diameter of the fetal renal pelvis (PD) and kidney (KD) provides useful information on the degree of hydronephrosis. A PD of 5–9 mm and a PD:KD ratio of less than 0.5 in the absence of rounded calyces is usually physiological. A PD of 10 mm or more and a PD:KD ratio of greater than 0.5 is usually pathological, particularly in the presence of rounded calyces. Hydronephrosis should only be diagnosed in the presence of calyceal dilatation.

Bladder Distention and Pyelectasis in Male Fetuses

- The presence of OH progressive bladder wall thickening and dilated posterior urethra is most suggestive of posterior urethral valves.
- The presence of patent urachus is most suggestive of prune belly syndrome.
- The presence of pyelectasis and megacystis without additional AF, bladder, urethral or renal abnormalities is most suggestive of vesicoureteral reflux, PUJ obstruction or non-refluxing non-obstructive megacystis-megaureter.

NB There is, however, overlap of some of the above findings between posterior urethral valves, prune belly syndrome, vesicoureteric reflux and non-refluxing non-obstructive megacystis-megaureter.

Further Reading

Anderson N, Clautice-Engle T, Allan R et al (1995) Detection of obstructive uropathy in the fetus predictive value of sonographic measurements of renal pelvic diameter at various gestational ages. *AJR* 164(3): 719–723.

Benacerraf BR, Madell J, Estroll JA et al (1990) Fetal pyelectasis: a possible association with Down's syndrome. *Obstet Gynecol* 76: 58–60.

Montemarano H, Bulas DI, Rushton G & Selby D (1998) Bladder distension and pyelectasis in male fetuses: causes, comparison and contrasts. *J Ultrasound Med* 17: 743–749.

Seed JW (1998) Borderline genitourinary tract abnormalities. *Seminars in Ultrasound CT and MRI* 19: 347–354.

Developmental Consequences of Fetal Urethral Obstruction

Hydronephrosis	• Cystic renal dysplasia
	• Renal failure
	• Urinomas/fetal ascites
	• Secondary reflux
Oligohydramnios	• Potter facies
	• Hypoplastic lungs
	• Flexion contractures
Megacystis	Abdominal muscle deficiency – 'prune belly'

Non-Visualized Fetal Urinary Bladder

Evacuated bladder

The fetal bladder is reliably seen by 12 weeks but before 16 weeks it may be empty for quite long periods. The fetal bladder normally empties every 30–45 minutes. During the course of an ultrasound study the bladder size may increase, or voiding may be observed as the urine streams into the amniotic fluid. Non-visualization over a 30-minute period justifies suspicion and re-examination to confirm non-visualization. Assessment of AF is an essential part of the examination of the bladder to confirm or refute urinary tract abnormalities but is not helpful before 18–20 weeks of gestation as AF is derived from other sources even in the case of bilateral renal agenesis.

Bilateral renal agenesis

Bilateral renal agenesis (Potter's syndrome) has an incidence of 1 in 3000–4000. It is incompatible with life and most affected infants die within a few hours of birth because of pulmonary hypoplasia caused by OH. Low-set ears, hypertelorism, beak nose and limb deformity may occur as a result of OH.

Bilateral severe renal dysplasia

The majority of cases of multicystic renal dysplasia are unilateral, but when bilateral the condition is fatal, with OH and pulmonary hypoplasia.

Bilateral severe renal hypoplasia

Renal hypoplasia may be unilateral or bilateral and the small kidney may be difficult to locate. The contralateral kidney may be hypertrophied, but if it is small then there may be OH. Renal hypoplasia may also be associated with other anomalies.

Bladder extrophy	This is a rare malformation occurring once in 50 000 births. The bladder is exposed on the abdominal wall and there is diastasis of the symphysis pubis. If the mucosa of the posterior bladder wall protrudes through the abdominal defect it may cause a prominence on the abdominal wall. Free communication between the bladder and amniotic cavity prevents bladder distention.
Bilateral PUJ obstruction	Approximately 10–30% of PUJ obstructions are bilateral but involvement is usually asymmetric and severe bilateral obstruction is rare. When bilateral PUJ obstruction is severe there will be OH, which may cause pulmonary hypoplasia. Paradoxically PH may also occur in up to 25% of cases.
Unilateral PUJ with contralateral renal agenesis/dysplastic kidney	Rarely unilateral PUJ obstruction may be associated with contralateral renal agenesis or multicystic dysplastic kidney, both of which increase the significance of the PUJ obstruction.
Evisceration of bladder in gastroschisis	With larger anterior abdominal wall defects, the stomach as well as the urinary bladder (and in the female fetus the adnexae) may be extruded into the amniotic cavity. The characteristic sonographic feature of gastroschisis is the observation of free loops of bowel floating in the amniotic fluid as early as 14 weeks of gestation.
Herniation of urinary bladder in LBWC	The limb-body wall complex is a severe malformation with multiple system anomalies. The lateral body wall defect may involve the thorax, the abdomen or both. There is visceral evisceration through the fetal trunk defects. The eviscerated organs form a complex mass, with the individual organs non-recognizable.

Further Reading

Clautice-Engle T, Pretorius DH & Budoroick NE (1991) Significance of non-visualisation of the fetal urinary bladder. *J Ultrasound Med* 10: 615–618.

Extremely Large Fetal Urinary Bladder (Megacystis)

Posterior urethral valves	PUV are the most common cause of urinary tract obstruction and end-stage renal failure in boys occurring in 1 in 5000–8000 males. The most common type extends distally from the veramontanum and divides into two membranes that run along the anterolateral wall of the urethra. Increased pressure from obstruction causes elongation and dilatation of the posterior urethra. Other types of PUV running proximally or distally and related to the veramontanum have been described. US reveals signs of urinary tract obstruction, bladder wall thickening (>2 mm), +/– dilatation of the posterior urethra, bright echogenic lines representing the urethral valves, dilatation of the renal collecting system, tortuosity of the dilated ureters, urinoma due to rupture of calyces and urinary ascites may occur. The combination of a dilated thick walled bladder and dilated posterior urethra gives the US appearance of a 'keyhole.' OH in the presence of massive bladder dilatation usually indicates a poor prognosis.
Urethral atresia/absence of urethra	The kidneys may be hydronephrotic or dysplastic and echogenic. There is massive dilatation of the bladder, which occupies most of the fetal abdomen. OH is always associated.
Megacystis-microcolon-intestinal hypoperistalsis syndrome	MMIHS is a rare congenital anomaly. The syndrome consists of intestinal malrotation, functional intestinal obstruction, microcolon and large non-obstructed urinary bladder. The last is a striking and constant finding on prenatal ultrasonography. OH may be observed in the second and early third trimester. The fetal megacystis is usually accompanied by upper renal tract dilatation. In later pregnancy dilated loops of bowel may be demonstrated.

Prune belly syndrome	This syndrome is characterized by severe deficiency of the abdominal wall musculature associated with gross dilatation of the bladder and ureters. This may follow resolution of urinary ascites.
Caudal regression syndrome	This is a rare syndrome characterized by vertebral agenesis of varying degree and a wide variety of associated anomalies. The vertebral agenesis can vary from partial agenesis to total agenesis of the lumbosacral spine. The syndrome is strongly associated with maternal insulin-dependent diabetes. The incidence is 200 times higher in diabetic than non-diabetic pregnancies. There is a constellation of CVS, GIT, CNS, genitourinary and musculo-skeletal defects.

Further Reading

Cohen HL, Zinn HL & Patel A (1998) Prenatal sonographic diagnosis of posterior urethral valves: identification of valves and thickening of the posterior urethral wall. *JCU* 26: 366–370.

Stamm E, King G & Thickman D (1991) Megacystis-microcolon-intestinal hypoperistalsis syndrome: prenatal identification in siblings and review of the literature. *J Ultrasound Med* 10: 599–602.

Fetal Genital Anomalies

Fetal gender and the external genitalia can usually be seen on ultrasound if the fetal position is suitable and oligohydramnios is not present. Accurate fetal determination is possible >20 weeks gestation in 94–100% of fetuses. Gender determination is of particular importance in X-linked genetic disorders. Fetal testes remain intra-abdominal structures until after 28 weeks gestation.

Cloacal dysgenesis	This may occur as an isolated lesion or as a part of a spectrum of anomalies involving multiple organ systems. Sonographic diagnostic clues suggesting cloacal dysgenesis include the presence of a single, thick-walled septated cyst within the pelvis in the absence of a recognizable fetal bladder. There may also be bilateral hydronephrosis, renal cysts, OH, transient fetal ascites, IUGR and sacral agenesis. The affected fetus is always a female.
Congenital hydrocele	Hydrocele may be either (1) communicating with the peritoneal cavity, or (2) non-communicating; repeat sonographic examination in the latter shows no change in the size of the fluid collection in the scrotum, unlike communicating hydrocele which may change in size. Consecutive scans showing a change in scrotal volume may also raise the possibility of the presence of an inguinal hernia. Hydroceles without evidence of fetal ascites usually resolve spontaneously. Hydrocele is relatively common in the third trimester, and in the absence of other anomalies is regarded as a physiological phenomenon, which resolves spontaneously.

Undescended testes	Fetal gender determination is highly accurate in the 2nd and 3rd trimester. Cryptorchidism occurs in 3% of full-term males – unilateral/bilateral. The finding of cryptorchidism may occur in an otherwise normal fetus, but may be associated with severe multiple congenital abnormalities. The finding may lead to incorrect sex assignment due to masculinization of female genitalia.
Ambiguous genitalia	Seen when normal male or female anatomy is not apparent.
Megaurethra	The dilated urethra is seen as a fluid-filled tube within the penis. Dilated urethra can occur with other disorders such as the prune belly syndrome, renal agenesis, renal hypoplasia, imperforate anus and congenital heart disease. The condition presents with a cystic mass placed between the fetal legs associated with a large urinary bladder and hydronephrosis.
Hypospadius	Hypospadius is a congenital abnormality in which the urethral meatus is abnormally placed – opening on the ventral penile surface proximal to the site of normal meatal opening. Hypospadius may form an isolated anomaly or may occur as a part of several well-defined syndromes – Optiz–Frias syndrome, Smith–Lemli–Optiz and Nager syndrome. US: The fetal phallus appears abnormally short, blunt-ended or curved with a bulbous distal end of the penis and cleft within the penis. There may be features of the associated syndromes.

Hydrometrocolpos and urogenital sinus	Usually caused by an imperforate hymen, which commonly becomes apparent at puberty. Exceptionally hydrometrocolpos may occur in a fetus when it is usually associated with a urogenital sinus or cloacal malformation. A urogenital sinus is caused when there is a common opening for the urinary bladder and vagina. With a urogenital sinus the rectum opens normally. The urogenital sinus commonly obstructs causing dilatation of the vagina and/or the urinary bladder. US: midline pelvic cyst/complex mass that displaces the bladder anteriorly often associated with hydronephrosis, cystic renal dysplasia and OH. The cyst may be so large as to fill the whole abdomen.
Urethral atresia	Urethral atresia usually causes a complete urethral obstruction causing massive bladder dilatation, which may fill the whole of the abdomen so as to compress not only intra-abdominal organs but also thoracic structures. There is OH. The prognosis is extremely poor.

Further Reading

Benacerraf BR, Bromley B (1998) Sonographic finding of undescended testes in fetuses at 35-40 weeks: significance and outcome. *JCU* 26: 69-71.

Benacerraf BR, Saltzman OH, Mandell J et al (1989) Sonographic diagnosis of abnormal fetal genitalia. *J Ultrasound Med* 8: 613-617.

Cooper C, Mahony BS, Bowie JD et al (1985) Prenatal ultrasound diagnosis of ambiguous genitalia. *J Ultrasound Med* 4: 433-436.

Fisk NM, Dhillon HK, Ellis CE et al (1990) Antenatal diagnosis of megalourethra in a fetus with prune belly syndrome. *JCU* 18: 124-128.

Lande IM & Hamilton EF (1986) The antenatal sonographic visualisation of cloacal dysgenesis. *J Ultrasound Med* 5: 275-278.

Petrikovsky BM, Walzok MP, D'Addaris PF et al (1988) Fetal cloacal anomalies. Prenatal sonographic findings and differential diagnosis. *Obstet Gynecol* 72: 464.

Pretorius DH, Halstead MJ, Abels W et al (1998) Hydrocele identified prenatally: common physiological phenomenon. *J Ultra Med* 17: 49-52.

Sides D, Goldstein RB, Baskin L, Kleiner BC (1996) Prenatal diagnosis of hypospadius. *J Ultra Med* 15: 741-746.

Fetal Suprarenal Masses

Adrenal hemorrhage

More common perinatally but has been reported in utero as an anechoic mass showing spontaneous regression over time. The incidence of adrenal hemorrhage is 1.7 per 1000 births at autopsy and 1.9 per 1000 births on neonatal US. The incidence of antenatal adrenal hemorrhage is not known. US diagnosis depends on the timing of the examination, in the first hours an adrenal hemorrhage appears echogenic but later becomes hypoechoic as adrenal hematoma diminishes, its borders become more echoic, the central hypoechoic component gradually disappears. Eventually a normal-sized adrenal gland with a rim of calcification may remain in the infant. The US appearances of prenatal adrenal hemorrhage do not always follow the typical course and neuroblastoma and adrenal hemorrhage may co-exist. An adrenal mass that changes on serial scans from cystic to semisolid is frequently adrenal hemorrhage.

Simple adrenal cysts

These have been reported as well-defined anechoic masses resolving spontaneously in the early neonatal period. There was no associated mass or calcification.

Adrenal cyst mimics

Renal cysts, hydronephrotic upper moiety of a duplex renal system and necrotic Wilms' tumor may mimic adrenal cysts. A post-natal follow up sonogram should resolve the issue.

Adrenal neuroblastoma | Rare but neuroblastomas account for the majority of antenatal tumors, frequently producing extensive metastases before birth. Typically there is a mixed cystic/solid suprarenal mass, cystic change may be the predominant feature. The tumor is most often cystic, right-sided and diagnosed in the 3rd trimester. Calcification is present in a small percentage. The tumors metastasize to the liver, marrow and bones. Liver metastases can be diagnosed prenatally. The tumor may grow rapidly. PH and solid neck masses (metastases) have been reported.

Other adrenal cysts | These may be lymphangiomatous, angiomatous retention cysts or cysts within an adenoma. They do not involute spontaneously. These cysts have been noted in infants but have not been reported in utero.

Neuroblastoma in situ | This is a benign lesion said to occur in 1.5% of normal newborns. The mass may occur in the fetus and is more commonly solid or complex rather than cystic. The lesion either resolves spontaneously or matures into normal adrenal tissue. Usually microscopic and therefore not seen.

Pulmonary sequestration | Subdiaphragmatic extralobar pulmonary sequestration usually presents as an echogenic mass, is left-sided and can be identified in the second trimester.

Differential Diagnosis of Antenatal Adrenal Hemorrhage

- Neuroblastoma
- Wilms tumour
- Adrenal cyst
- Adrenal abscess
- Adrenocortical cysts
- Adrenal nodular hyperplasia
- Duplication of renal pelvis
- Pulmonary sequestration
- Hepatic cysts
- Choledochal cysts
- Ovarian cysts
- Enteric cysts

Further Reading

Atkinson GO, Asatari GS, Lorenzo RL et al (1986) Cystic neuroblastoma in infants: radiographic and pathologic features. *AJR* 146: 113.

Curtis MR, Mooney DP, Vaccaro TJ et al (1997) Prenatal ultrasound characterisation of suprarenal mass: distinction between neuroblastoma and subdiaphragmatic extralobar pulmonary sequestration. *J Ultra Med* 16: 75-83.

Fang S-B, Lee H-C, Sheu J-C et al (1999) Prenatal sonographic detection of adrenal hemorrhage confirmed by post-natal surgery. *JCU* 27: 206-209.

Giulian BB, Chag CCN & Oss BS (1986) Prenatal ultrasonographic diagnosis of fetal adrenal neuroblastoma. *JCU* 14: 225.

Gotah T, Adachi Y, Nounaka D et al (1989) Adrenal hemorrhage in the newborn with evidence of bleeding in utero. *J Urol* 141: 1145.

Morganli VJ & Anderson NG (1991) Simple adrenal cysts in fetus, resolving spontaneously in neonate. *J Ultrasound Med* 10: 521-524.

Shen M-R, Lin Y-S, Huang S-C & Chou C-Y (1997) Rapid growth of fetal abdominal mass: a case report of congenital neuroblastoma. *JCU* 25: 39-42.

Strouse PJ, Bowerman RA & Schlesinger AE (1995) Antenatal sonographic findings of fetal adrenal hemorrhage. *JCU* 23: 442-446.

Fetal Musculoskeletal System

Limb Reduction Nomenclature

Achiria	Absence of hands.
Achiropody	Absence of hands and feet.
Acromelia	Distal limb shortening, especially hands/feet.
Adactyly	Absence of fingers or toes (ectrodactyly).
Amelia	Absence of an extremity (ectromelia).
Apodia	Absence of feet.
Hemimelia	Absence of limb below elbow or knee.
Mesomelia	Shortening of middle segments (forearm or lower leg).
Micromelia	Shortened limbs.
Phocomelia	Deficient proximal and midlimbs with preservation of distal limb (seal flipper deformity).
Radial paraxial hemimelia	Aplasia or hypoplasia of the radius and thumb associated with clubbed hand.
Rhizomelia	Shortening of proximal limb segments.
Synbrachydactyly	Short fused digits.
Ulnar paraxial hemimelia	Aplasia or hypoplasia of the ulna or ulnar digits.

Short-Limbed Dwarfism

Achondroplasia

Genetic disorder, endochondral bone formation with autosomal dominant mode of inheritance. Achondroplasia may be inherited in a homozygous or heterozygous manner. Heterozygous disease is a common skeletal dysplasia – 1:2600 births, 80% are due to spontaneous mutation causing rhizomelic shortening, large head with frontal bossing, depressed nasal bridge, short trident hands and lumber lordosis. Mental and sexual development and life span is normal. The homozygous disease is lethal due to respiratory difficulties from thoracic constriction. Risk: one parent heterozygous: low: 1:50 000 (0.002%). Risk: both parents heterozygous 25%. Prenatal distinction between homozygous and heterozygous disease is important so that a well-informed decision can be made regards continuation of pregnancy.

Achondroplasia (homozygous)

Parents will both be heterozygotes. Rhizomelic micromelia, normal trunk length, ± cloverleaf skull. These cases are lethal. Lung hypoplasia is a major cause of mortality (due to thoracic narrowing). Noticeable disproportion between skull dimensions/BPD and limb lengths. The discrepancy between femoral length and BPD is noted as early as 13 weeks gestation. The femoral length decreases to below third percentile at 14.0–16.5 weeks BPD age (mean 15.6 weeks ± 1.1; 95% confidence interval 13.4, 17.8 weeks). Thus establishment of femoral growth curves in the second trimester with serial US scans enables prenatal distinction between homozygous and heterozygous disease.

Achondroplasia
(heterozygous)

Changes less severe, short limbs, thorax and abdomen narrow. Increased fetal head circumference and BPD, protuberant forehead, narrow interpedicular distance in the spine. Heterozygous disease may not be recognized until late in the second trimester (>24–28 weeks), early sonography being normal. There is rhizomelic limb (proximal long bones more affected) shortening.

Achondrogenesis type I

Autosomal recessive lethal dwarfism (Parenti–Fraccara, type 1A – Houston–Harris, type 1B – Fraccara – 20%). Both endochondral and membranous ossification are affected – calvarium, spine as well as long bones, frequent rib fractures. Severe short-limbed dwarfism, poorly ossified skull and rest of the skeleton. Marked chest narrowing, the head is not enlarged relative to the trunk. PH is usually present.

Achondrogenesis

Langer–Saldino (80%) autosomal recessive. Less severe than type 1 endochondral ossification affected – variable calcification of calvarium and spine, no rib fractures but lethal short-limbed dwarfism of long bone type. The head is large relative to the rest of the body, prominent skin folds over a short neck, small chest, distended abdomen with FH, short limbs are held extended away from the body.

Chondroectodermal
dysplasia

(Ellis–Van Creveld syndrome). Autosomal recessive with variable expression. Severely shortened ribs, short limbs, narrow thorax, polydactyly, CHD (50% have a large ASD), postaxial hexadactyly. The size of thorax is particularly striking when compared with the abdomen and head.

Asphyxiating thoracic
dystrophy

(Jeune's syndrome). Autosomal recessive, extremely narrow thorax ± rhizomelic short-limb dwarfism ± polydactyly ± renal dysplasia (renal cysts).

Osteogenesis imperfecta type IIa	Autosomal dominant, usually lethal; thin skull vault which may collapse, limbs short, thickened and angulated due to multiple fractures.
Osteogenesis imperfecta type I, III, IV	Autosomal dominant or sporadic; has normal body proportions and fractures with normal bone lengths.
Hypophosphatasia (congenital)	Congenital hypophosphatasia is an autosomal recessive disorder, which in the homozygous causes severe deficiency of alkaline phosphatase and increased excretion of phosphoethanolamine. There is severe demineralization of bones. Incidence – 1:100 000 births. Four types are described: neonatal (congenital), juvenile, adult and latent, the latter is a mild form and is thought to be autosomal dominant. US: short-limbed dwarfism, thin delicate bones with reduced echogenicity. First trimester chorionic sampling with alkaline phosphatase assay may establish the diagnosis.
Metatrophic dysplasia	Varied inheritance; narrow thorax, kyphoscoliosis relatively long trunk ± tail-like appendage over the sacrum.
Roberts' syndrome	(Pseudothalidomide syndrome) Autosomal recessive with variable expression, tetraphocomelia, midline facial cleft. The chromosomes show a classical abnormality with the centromere region being fluffy.
Diastrophic dysplasia	Autosomal recessive, multiple contractures, hitchhiker's thumb (more muscle mass than arthrogryposis).

Short rib-polydactyly
syndrome

Type I	(Saldino–Noonan) Autosomal recessive. Severely shortened ribs/narrow thorax, short limbs, polydactyly, CVS and genital anomalies, polycystic kidney and pointed metaphysis (important differentiating feature).
Type II	(Majewski) Short limbs, narrow thorax, polydactyly, CVS anomalies, polycystic kidneys, genital anomalies, disproportionately short tibia*, cleft lip and palate*. (*Important differentiating feature.)
Type III	(Naumoff) Short limbs, narrow thorax, polydactyly, CVS and genital anomalies. The metaphysis may be wide with marginal spurs.

NB Large polycystic kidneys, occipital encephalocele, microcephaly or polydactyly may be associated with any type of short rib-polydactyly syndrome.

Spondyloepiphyseal dysplasia congenita	Autosomal dominant with variable expression, short bowed femora, short spine and trunk (delayed ossification centers, calcaneus and talus).
Camptomelic dysplasia	Anterior bowing of the lower extremity long bones, anomalies of cervical and thoracic spine with spinal scoliosis and hypoplastic or absent scapulas.
Thanatophoric dysplasia	Occurs sporadically, represents the most common lethal skeletal dysplasia; 14% have a cloverleaf skull (this may be transmitted in an autosomal recessive manner), marked narrowing of the thorax, marked micromelia, soft tissues of limbs may be thickened, enlargement of the head (± prominent forehead), occasional hydrocephalus, PH, more common in male fetuses.

Fibrochondrogenesis	Autosomal recessive; thin skull vault, poorly echogenic, may be difficult to identify, collapsed sutures occasionally seen, limbs short and thin, ribs thin and poorly visualized, spine poorly mineralized and poorly visualized. Widened metaphyses.
Chondrodysplasia punctata (rhizomelic type)	Severe micromelia of humeri and femora, multiple joint contractures, vertebral body dorsal and ventral ossification separated by a cartilaginous bar.
Kniest's dysplasia	Autosomal dominant kyphoscoliosis, short trunk, broad thorax, prognosis usually good. Widened metaphyses.
Mesomelic and acromesomelic dysplasia	Autosomal recessive/autosomal dominant; micromelia of middle or distal segments, distribution of shortening differentiates from lethal syndromes.

Differential Diagnosis of Chondrodysplasia Punctata

- Rhizomelic chondrodysplasia punctata
- Non-rhizomelic chondrodysplasia punctata (Conradi Hunermann, Tibia-metacarpal type of chondrodysplasia punctata)
- Trisomy 18
- Trisomy 21
- Zellweger syndrome
- Vitamin K reductase deficiency
- Drugs: warfarin, phenytoin, phenprocoumon, acenocoumarol, fetal alcohol syndrome, and phenacetin intoxication

Short-Rib Dwarfism

- Thoracic asphyxiating dystrophy (Jeune's syndrome) – often cystic renal disease
- Thanatophoric dysplasia

Short-rib-polydactyly syndrome (SRP)

- SPR 1 (Saldino–Noonan) – short ribs, marked micromelia and absent vertebrae
- SPR II (Majewski) – similar to type I but normal vertebrae and cleft lip
- SPR III (Verma–Naumoff) – 50% males, often no polydactyly, ball in cone end of bones
- SPR IV (Beemer-Langer) – same as type II except no polydactyly

Further Reading

Benacerraf BR (1993) Prenatal sonographic diagnosis of short rib-polydactyly syndrome. Type II Majewski type. *J Ultrasound Med* 12: 552-555.

Bulas DI, Stern HJ, Rosenbaum KN et al (1994) Variable prenatal appearance of osteogenesis imperfecta. *J Ultrasound Med* 13(6): 419-427.

Delonge M & Rouse GA (1990) Prenatal diagnosis of hypophosphatasia. *J Ultrasound Med* 9: 113-117.

Gembruch U, Hansmann M & Modisch HJ (1985) Early prenatal diagnosis of short rib-polydactyly (SRP) syndrome type I (Majewski) by ultrasound in a case of risk. *Prenat Diagn* 5: 357.

Goncalves L & Jeanty P (1994) Fetal biometry of skeletal dysplasias: multicentric study. *J Ultrasound Med* 13: 977-980.

Hertzberg BS, Kliewer MA, Deker M et al (1999) Antenatal ultrasonographic diagnosis of rhizomelic chondrodysplasia punctata. *J Ultra Med* 18: 715-718.

Meizner I & Bar-Ziv J (1985) Prenatal ultrasonic diagnosis of short rib-polydactyly syndrome (SRPS) type III. A case report and proposed approach to the diagnosis of SRPS and related conditions. *JCU* 13:284.

Patel MD & Filly RA (1995) Homozygous achondroplasia: US distinction between homozygous, heterozygous and unaffected fetuses in the second trimester. *Radiology* 196(2): 541-545.

Pretorius DH, Rumack CM, Manco-Johnson ML et al (1986) Specific skeletal dysplasias in utero: sonographic diagnosis. *Radiology* 159: 237.

Sanders RC, Greyson-Fleg RT, Hogge WA et al (1994) Osteogenesis imperfecta and camptomelic dysplasia. *J Ultrasound Med* 13(9): 691-700.

Tongsong T & Chanprapaph P (2000) Prenatal sonographic diagnosis of Ellis-van Creveld syndrome. *JCU* 28: 38-41.

Tongsong T, Srisomboon J & Sudasna J (1995) Prenatal diagnosis of Langer-Saldingo achondrogenesis. *JCU* 23: 56-58.

Tongsong T, Sirichotiyakul S & Siriangkul S (1995) Prenatal diagnosis of congenital hypophosphatasia. *JCU* 23: 52–55.

Tongsong T, Chanprapaph P & Thongpadunqro JT (1999) Prenatal sonographic findings associated with asphyxiating thoracic dystrophy. *J Ultra Med* 18: 573–576.

Osteochondrodysplasias with Normal Body Proportions

Osteogenesis imperfecta (type I, III and IV)	± Multiple fractures with normal or nearly normal bone lengths.
Cleidocranial dysostosis	Autosomal dominant; 30% occur by spontaneous mutation. Clavicular hypoplasia/aplasia, brachycephaly with increased BPD and frontal bossing.
Otopalatodigital syndrome	X-linked with minor manifestation. Camptodactyly, hypoplasia of fibulas, phalanges, metacarpals/metatarsals, syndactyly, cleft palate.
Larsen syndrome	Defect of collagen formation including multiple disorders of the joints and cardiac anomalies, multiple joint dislocations, abnormal facies, facial clefting, hemi- and butterfly vertebrae, hypoplasia of proximal radius, short thumb, talipes, hypertelorism ± kyphoscoliosis. Some cases are familial – both autosomal dominant and recessive, some cases are lethal but generally the prognosis is favorable after aggressive orthopedic management. US: multiple joint dislocations, abnormal position of legs and knees and club feet, abnormally depressed nasal bridge, hypertelorism and prominent forehead and cleft lip.
Osteopetrosis congenita	Hepatosplenomegaly. Requires radiological confirmation.
Ectrodactyly-ectodermal dysplasia-cleft palate syndrome	Autosomal dominant, ectrodactyly (lobster claw deformity), cleft lip and palate. Additional findings include urinary tract involvement, conductive hearing loss and atresia of lacrimal duct.

Caudal regression syndrome	Absence of sacrum associated with talipes, absent limb elements, flexion contractures, sirenomelia, anorectal atresia, intestinal malrotation, patent cloaca, TOF, gastroschisis, duodenal atresia, renal agenesis, multicystic dysplastic kidneys, duplication/absence of genitalia, CHD, pulmonary hypoplasia, DWM and hydrocephalus. There is a strong association with maternal insulin-dependent diabetes.

Further Reading

Hertzberg BS, Kliewer MA, Paulyson-Nunez K (2000) Lethal multiple pterygium syndrome. *J Ultra Med* 19: 657–660.

Lewit N, Batino S, Groisman GM et al (1995) Early prenatal diagnosis of Larsen's syndrome by transvaginal sonography. *J Ultrasound Med* 14: 627–629.

Mahoney BS (1994) The fetal musculo-skeletal system. In: Callen PW (ed.) *Ultrasonography in Obstetrics and Gynecology,* 3rd edn, pp 254–290. Philadelphia: WB Saunders.

Tongsong T, Wanapirak C, Pongsatha S & Suldasana J (2000) Prenatal sonographic diagnosis of Larson syndrome. *J Ultra Med* 19: 419–421.

Twickler D, Budorick N, Pretorius DH et al (1993) Caudal regression versus sirenomelia: sonographic clues. *J Ultrasound Med* 12(6): 323–330.

Widened Metaphyses

Metatrophic dysplasia	Narrow thorax, kyphoscoliosis, relatively long trunk ± tail-like appendage over the sacrum.
Weissenbacher–Zweymuller phenotype syndrome	Micrognathia, rhizomelic-type shortening of the limbs, widening of metaphyses, particularly femora and humeri.
Kniest's dysplasia	Kyphoscoliosis, short trunk and broad thorax.
Fibrochondrogenesis	Autosomal recessive (rare), lethal short-limbed dwarfism; undermineralized skull, soft tissue edema, platyspondyly, broad metaphyses. Associated anomalies; omphalocele, cleft palate, small abnormal-shaped ears.
Short-rib polydactyly syndrome type III	Short limbs, narrow thorax, polydactyly, CVS and genital anomalies, wide metaphyses with marginal spurs.
Dyssegmental dysplasia	Autosomal recessive, rare; micrognathia, cleft palate, narrow chest, broad metaphyses, short tubular bones, encephalocele, hydrocephalus, ear abnormalities and CHD.

Further Reading

Aleck KA et al (1987) Dyssegmental dysplasias. *Am J Med Genet* 27: 295–312.

Colavita N, Kozlowski K (1984) Neonatal death dwarfism: A new form. *Pediatr Radiol* 14: 451–452.

Kelly TE et al (1982) The Weissenbacher Zweymuller syndrome. *Am J Med Genet* 11: 113–119.

Whitley CB et al (1984) Fibrochondrogenesis. *Am J Med Genet* 19: 265–275.

Syndromes Associated with Radial Hypoplasia/Aplasia

Turner's syndrome	Associated with radial hypoplasia/aplasia. Cystic hygroma often seen.
Roberts' syndrome	(Pseudothalidomide syndrome) Autosomal recessive; tetraphocomelia, cleft lip/palate, absent thumbs (thumbs sometimes present) associated with multiple dysmorphic features and malformation.
Holt–Oram syndrome	Autosomal dominant; thumb and terminal upper-limb defects, upper-limb abnormality typically on the left side and range for hypoplasia of the thumb to phocomelia. Hypoplasia of the first metacarpal and radius, defects of fibula, humerus, clavicles, scapulae and sternum. Cardiac defects include secundum type ASD, other cardiac abnormalities include VSD, transposition, tetralogy of Fallot, Ebstein anomaly reported once.
Fanconi anemia	Autosomal recessive; terminal limb osseous defects, absent thumbs, renal anomalies.
Amniotic band syndrome	Asymmetric slash defects involving limb, face, head and trunk; a band may be seen in relation to the defect.
VACETRAL association	
TAR syndrome	(Thrombocytopenia – absent radius syndrome) Autosomal recessive; absent radius, commonly associated with CHD.

Fetal valproate syndrome	Valproate, a drug used in epilepsy, has been associated with a characteristic facial phenotype, which may not be detectable on antenatal ultrasound but other features of the syndrome such as radial aplasia, CHD, CNS (neural tube defects) and other skeletal anomalies are readily identified.
Levy–Hollister syndrome	(Lacrimoauriculodentodigital syndrome) Autosomal dominant; associated with malformed ears, beak-like nose, radial aplasia, digital and renal anomalies.
Baller–Gerold syndrome	? Autosomal recessive; associated with craniosynostosis, radial aplasia/hypoplasia, aplasia/hypoplasia of thumbs, missing phalanges, CHD, crossed renal ectopia and vertebral anomalies.
Seckel's syndrome	Autosomal recessive associated with severe IUGR, microcephaly, prominent beaked nose, micrognathia, bird-head profile – thus bird-headed dwarfism. Other features include clindactyly of fifth digits, absence of phalangeal epiphysis, simian crease, dislocation of radial head with hypoplasia of the proximal end of radius, 11 ribs and a small cerebellum. Most or all of the morphological features of the syndrome may be seen on US.
Trisomy 18	See page 341.
Goldenhar syndrome	
Aase syndrome	The condition comprises hypoplastic anemia as in Fanconi anemia but unlike the latter the thumb is triphalangeal.
Nager acrofacial dysostosis	An autosomal recessive disorder, which comprises micrognathia, cleft lip, radial and ulnar hypoplasia and absence of the fifth digits in the hands and feet.

Radial club-hand and cleft lip syndrome

Radial club-hand abnormalities have been described in association with chromosomal anomalies such as trisomies 18 and 21 and deletion of the long arm of chromosome 13 and ring formation of chromosome 4.

Further Reading

Bowerman RA (1995) Anomalies of the fetal skeleton: sonographic findings. *AJR* 164: 973–977.

Featherstone LS, Sherman SJ & Quigg MH (1996) Prenatal diagnosis of Seckel syndrome. *J Ultra Med* 15: 85–88.

Hedberg VA & Pipton JM (1989) Thrombocytopenia with absent radii. A review of 100 cases. *Am J Pediatr Hematol Oncol* 10: 51.

Hirose K, Kojanagi T, Hara K et al (1988) Antenatal ultrasound diagnosis of the femur-fibula-ulna syndrome. *J Clin Ultrasound* 16: 199.

Tongsong T & Chanprapaph P (2000) Prenatal sonographic diagnosis of Holt–Oram syndrome. *JCU* 28: 98–100.

Ylagan LR & Budovick NE (1994) Radial ray aplasia in utero: a prenatal finding associated with valproic acid exposure. *J Ultrasound Med* 13: 408–411.

Short Femurs in the Fetus

Artifact   Foreshortening of femur. Wrong dates.

Causes of short limb dysplasia

- Artifact. Shadowing by another osseous structure.
- Achondroplasia. See page 337.
- Osteogenesis imperfecta. See page 338.
- Short rib-polydactyly. See page 339.
- Chondroectodermal dysplasia. See page 337.
- Proximal femoral focal deficiency. Sonography reveals unequal femur lengths (bilateral in 10–15%). Normal fetus with only one short femur has virtually no other differential diagnosis. Associated anomalies include intercalary hemimelias, tibial camptomelia, phocomelia of another limb, amelia, spinal dysraphism and microcephaly.
- Down's syndrome.
- Amniotic band syndrome. See page 347.
- Camptomelic dysplasia. See page 339.
- Achondrogenesis. See page 337.
- Seckel's syndrome. Microcephaly, prominent nose (beak-like), ocular hypertelorism, micrognathia, hypoplastic thumb, kyphoscoliosis, rhizomelic shortening of humeri and femora.
- Fibular hemimelia. Most common long bone defect, classic presentation: complete absence, marked AP bowing of tibia, marked talipes equinovalgus and absence of one or more lateral rays of the foot. Additionally ipsilateral short femur abnormalities of femoral head and neck. 50% associated with femoral focal deficiency and associated omphalocele has been reported twice. US: absent fibula and bowed tibia.

Further Reading

Camera G, Dedro D, Parodi M et al (1993) Antenatal ultrasonographic diagnosis of a proximal femoral focal deficiency. *J Ultrasound Med* 21: 475–479.

Caspi G (1990) Unilateral congenital short femur; a case report. *Prenat Diagn* 10: 67.

Golbus MS, Hall B, Filly RA et al (1977) Prenatal diagnosis of achondrogenesis. *J Pediatr* 91: 464–466.

Jeanty P & Kleiman G (1989) Proximal femoral focal deficiency. *J Ultrasound Med* 8: 639–642.

Jeanty P, Kirkpatrick C, Dramaix-Wilmet M et al (1981) Ultrasonic evaluation of fetal limb growth. *Radiology* 140: 165–168.

Kerat D & Timar IE (1988) Familial congenital short femur. Intrauterine detection and follow-up by ultrasound. *Orthop Rev* 27: 500.

O'Rahilly R (1951) Morphologic patterns in limb deficiencies and duplications. *Am J Anat* 80: 135.

Quennan TJ, O'Brien CD & Campbell S (1980) Ultrasound measurement of fetal limb bones. *Am J Obstet Gynecol* 138: 297–302.

Uffelman J, Woo BSR, Richards DS (2000) Prenatal diagnosis of bilateral fibular hemimelia. *J Ultra Med* 19: 341–344.

Anomalies Associated with Fetal Clubfoot

Fetal talipes not associated with OH is often seen with other fetal anomalies.

Chromosomal defects   Triploidy, trisomies 18, 13, 9, mosaic 20p, 4p, 9p, partial trisomy 10q, 13q, 18q XXXX and XXXY syndrome.

Skeletal dysplasias   Diastrophic dysplasia, osteogenesis imperfecta, Kniest's dysplasia, spondyloephiphyseal dysplasia congenita, metatrophic dysplasia, mesomelic dysplasia (Nievergelt type), chondrodysplasia punctata, Roberts' syndrome, Pena–Shokeir syndrome, Larsen's syndrome, arthrogryposis multiplex congenita, Ellis–van Creveld syndrome, Conradi–Hunermann and nail-patella syndromes.

Neural tube defects   Spina bifida/meningomyelocele and hydrocephalus.

Metabolic disorders   Homocystinuria, Hunter's syndrome, Ehlers–Danlos syndrome, gangliosidosis – generalized, Zellweger's syndrome.

Dysostoses   Femoral hypoplasia.

Teratogens   Aminopterin fetopathy.

Miscellaneous disorders   Aarskog's, Escobar's, Bloom's, Dubowitz's, Freeman–Sheldon, Hecht's, Meckel's, Noonan's, Mietens–Weber, Riley–Day, Schwartz–Jampel, Seckel's, tar syndromes and myotonic dystrophy.

Isolated

Further Reading

Hasimoto DE, Filly RA & Callan PW (1986) Sonographic diagnoses of clubfoot in utero. *J Ultrasound Med* 5: 81–85.

In Utero Contractures/Absent Limb/Joint Movement

Oligohydramnios
Adequate amniotic fluid is required to allow for normal development of fetal lungs and normal fetal movements. With diminution of amniotic fluid, postural defects such as a clubfoot may result.

Arthrogryposis multiplex
Usually associated with PH, extremities maintained in a fixed and rigid posture which remains unchanged from examination to examination.

Diastrophic dwarfism
See page 338.

Osteogenesis imperfecta
See pages 338, 344.

Pena–Shokeir syndrome
See page 357.

IUGR
In high-risk pregnancies with IUGR, fetal movement and fetal breathing movements may be reduced. Normally there are 10–16 discrete movements occurring in episodes of 30 minutes on real time sonography. Fetuses that spend less than 50% of their time breathing tend to have a poor prognosis.

Myelomeningocele
Clubfoot in meningomyelocele may be a manifestation of its neurologic effect in the lower limbs.

Trisomy 18
See page 341.

Mesomelic dysplasia
See page 340 (Nievergelt type).

Roberts' syndrome
See page 347 (Pseudothalidomide syndrome).

Chondrodysplasia punctata
See page 340.

Myotonic dystrophy	Autosomal dominant; reduced fetal movements, PH, hydrops fetalis, pleural effusions, joint contractures, tented upper lip, respiratory and feeding difficulty after birth.
Metatrophic dwarfism	See page 338.
Acrocephalosyndactyly (Apert type)	
Microcephaly	
Pterygium syndrome	PS produces contracture deformities from webs extending across limb joints. Popliteal PS is inherited in an autosomal dominant manner with variable expression and incomplete penetrance. Multiple PS on the other hand is inherited in an autosomal recessive manner and is a much more serious disease, causing webs involving the neck, axilla, elbow, knee and digits. US: limb contractures, absent fetal limb motion and cystic hygroma, hydrops, IUGR, there may be direct visualization of pterygia themselves and other ancillary findings.
Kleeblattschadel anomaly	

de Lange's syndrome	Multisystem disease (Brachmann de Lange) 1:10 000, most cases sporadic but both autosomal dominant and autosomal recessive inheritance has been implicated in rare cases. There is also considerable overlap with duplication 3q syndrome. There is prenatal and postnatal growth deficiency, characteristic facies, microbrachycephaly, micromelia, phocomelia, hemimelia, anomalies of digits, limb contractures with anomalies of GIT, hydrocephalus/cerebral ventricular dilatation, horse-shoe kidneys, diaphragmatic hernia, long lashes and abnormal facial profile. Although the clinical features of duplication 3q syndrome may be identical differentiation can easily be made. Duplication 3q syndrome is more often associated with craniosynostosis, cleft palate and renal abnormalities.
Kniest's syndrome	See page 340.
Focal femoral deficiency	See page 350.
Sacral agenesis	
Bilateral renal agenesis	Effects related to OH.
Harlequin fetus	Autosomal recessive lethal form of congenital ichthyosis characterized by massive overgrowth of keratin layer of fetal skin. Preterm birth is common, in severe form infants live only a few days. Prenatal diagnosis has been achieved by an in utero skin biopsy. US: fixed flexion of hands and open mouth.

In Utero Joint Dislocations and Hyperextensions

- Larsen syndrome
- Arthrogryposis multiplex congenita
- Pena–Shokier syndrome
- Trisomy 18
- Congenital myotonic dystrophy
- Non-lethal pterygium syndrome
- Lethal pterygium syndrome.

Further Reading

Baty BJ, Cubberley D, Morris C et al (1988) Prenatal diagnosis of distal arthrogryposis. *Am J Med Genet* 29: 501.

Camera G, Dodero D, Parodi M et al (1993) Antenatal ultrasonographic diagnosis of a proximal femoral focal deficiency. *JCU* 21: 475–476.

Cardwell MS (1987) Pena–Shokeir syndrome prenatal diagnosis by ultrasonography. *J Ultrasound Med* 6: 619-621.

Genkins SM, Hertzberg BS, Bowie JD et al (1989). Pena–Shokeir type I syndrome. In utero sonographic appearances. *JCU* 17: 56.

Hall JG (1986) Invited editorial comment. Analysis of Pena–Shokeir phenotype. *Am J Med Genet* 25: 99.

Lowey JA, Richards DG & Toi A (1987) In utero diagnosis of the caudal regression syndrome. Report of three cases. *JCU* 15: 469-474.

McMillan RH, Herbert GM, Davies WD et al (1985) Prenatal diagnosis of Pena–Shokeir syndrome type I. *Am J Med Genet* 21: 279.

Ranzini A, Day-Salvatore D, Farren-Chavez D et al (1997) Prenatal diagnosis of de Lange syndrome. *J Ultra Med* 16: 753-758.

Watson WJ, Mcbee CM (1995) Prenatal diagnosis of severe congenital ichthyosis (Harlequin fetus) by ultrasonography. *J Ultra Med* 14: 241-243.

Cysts in Fetal Subcutaneous Tissues

Klippel–Trenaunay syndrome

Sonography demonstrates peripheral and visceral vascular anomalies. The angiodysplastic lesions in the subcutaneous tissue may appear as cystic areas. Hemihypertrophy may be seen.

Subcutaneous lymphangiomas

The cystic spaces are usually less than 5 mm in diameter; hemihypertrophy/focal hypertrophy does not normally occur.

Hemangioma

Hemangiomas may occur as an isolated anomaly in the subcutaneous tissue unassociated with Klippel–Trenaunay–Weber syndrome. Color Doppler may demonstrate active flow within the cystic spaces.

Proteus syndrome

Hemi/focal hypertrophy, macrodactyly, subcutaneous cysts and intra-abdominal masses.

Hamartoma

These tumors, which may be cystic or complex, are known to occur in the neck, thorax or abdomen. A case of extensive vascular hamartomatosis involving the whole of the body has been described. The appearances were those of multiple subcutaneous cystic spaces.

Differential Diagnosis of Fetal Limb Swelling

Klippel–Trenaunay–Weber syndrome	Hypertrophy of one or occasionally more than one limb – may coincide with hemangiomatous involvement. The swelling usually involves the entire limb.
Lymphangioma	Malformation consisting of dilated lymphatic channels of various sizes lined by endothelium – fluid-filled vesicles or cysts of various sizes.
Congenital lymphedema	Classified into primary lymphedema and the hereditary form (Milroy's disease). The edema is usually confined to the lower limbs but may develop a chylothorax and chylous ascites. There is an association with Turner's (XO) syndrome.
Congenital fibrosarcoma	Congenital fibrosarcoma of the mediastinum (echogenic mass invading the sternum), of the neck (huge hypervascular tumor) and the leg have been reported antenatally. Fibrosarcoma of the limb presented with soft-tissue over-growth with overlying redundant skin but usually cause focal lesion rather than involvement of the whole limb.
Lipomatosis	Fatty tumors may infiltrate subcutaneous tissue or muscles, visceral involvement may occur. Rarely focal hypertrophy may occur secondary to lipomatous tumors.

Infantile myofibromatosis

Most common soft tissue tumor of infancy and early childhood, rarely encountered in newborns. The mortality rate is about 15%, prognosis depending upon visceral involvement, pulmonary involvement in particular has a poor prognosis. Without visceral involvement prognosis is good. Two types are described – solitary in skin, muscle, bone or subcutaneous tissues, multicentric type affecting the subcutaneous tissues only or subcutaneous musculoskeletal system and viscera. US: inhomogeneous moderately echogenic soft-tissue tumors.

Protruding Superficial Sacral Mass

- Lipoma
- Sacrococcygeal teratoma
- Spina bifida
- Lipomeningocele: lipoma of spinal cord uncommon 1:4000 live births. The tumor is skin covered and usually associated with spina bifida occulta. Some cases are associated with cloacal extrophy, asymmetry of the limbs and minor neurological deficit. Prenatal US: dysraphism, semisolid echogenic mass continuous with the sacral area and bulged posteriorly under the skin.

Further Reading

Arienzo R, Ricco CS & Romero F (1987) A very rare fetal malformation. The cutaneous widespread vascular hamartomatosis. *Am J Obstet Gynecol* 157: 1162.

Helin I & Persson PH (1985) Intra-abdominal cysts detected at prenatal ultrasound screening. *Helv Paediatr Acta* 40: 55.

Kubota A, Imano M, Yonekura T et al (1999) Infantile myofibromatosis of the triceps detected by prenatal sonography. *JCU* 27: 147–150.

Richards DS, Williamson CA, Crue AC & Hendrickson JE (1991) Prenatal sonographic findings in a fetus with proteus syndrome. *J Ultrasound Med* 10: 47–50.

Sharony R, Aviram R, Tohar M et al (2000) Prenatal sonographic deletion of a lipomeningocele as a sacral lesion. *JCU* 28: 150–152.

Suma V, Marini A, Gomba PG et al (1990) Giant hemangioma of the thigh: prenatal sonographic diagnosis. *JCU* 18: 421.

Tadmor OP, Ariel I, Robinowitz R et al (1998) Prenatal sonographic appearance of congenital fibrosarcoma. *JCU* 26: 276–279.

Warhit JM, Goldman MA, Sachs L et al (1983) Klippel–Trenaunay–Weber syndrome: Appearances in utero. *J Ultrasound Med* 2: 515.

PART 2

GYNECOLOGY

10

Pediatric and Adolescent Gynecology

Ovarian Size

At birth	1.5 × 0.3 × 0.25 cm.
After puberty	2.4-4.1 × 1.5-2.4 × 0.85-1.9 cm.
Ovarian volume	Length × width × depth × 0.52 ml (assuming the ovary is elliptical in shape).
Volume	Child - 1 ml Adult - 7-7.5 ml (normally <10 ml) Postmenopausal - 1.5-10 ml.

Before the menopause ovarian volume will obviously depend upon the number and size of developing follicles.

Further Reading

Haber HP & Mayar EL (1994) Ultrasound evaluation of uterine and ovarian size from birth to puberty. *Pediatric Radiol* 24(1): 11-13.

Uterine Measurements

Neonatal uterus

Average size: length 3.4 cm
                width 1.25 cm

NB The fetus is subject to the influence of maternal hormones and thus at birth the neonatal uterus has a similar configuration to the postpubertal uterus. The uterus involutes over the next few weeks. Intracavitary fluid is a common normal finding.

Prepubertal uterus

Average size: length 2–3.3 cm
                width 0.5–1 cm

NB At this stage the body and cervix of the uterus are of similar length, giving a body/cervix ratio of 1:1. After puberty the ratio increases to 2:1.

Puberty

Average size: length 5–8 cm
                width 1.6–3 cm

Uterine volume

Approximately length × width × breadth × 0.5.
Prepubertal: <2 ml.
Puberty: 25 ml.

Pregnancy

During pregnancy the uterus increases in size up to 30 times by muscle hypertrophy. After pregnancy it involutes but usually remains larger than before.

Uterine hypoplasia

Not usually evident until puberty. Causes include lack of estrogens, chromosomal anomalies and in utero exposure to diethylestilbestrol.

Further Reading

Haber HD & Mayer EI (1994) Ultrasound evaluation of uterine and ovarian size from birth to puberty. *Pediatr Radiol* 24(1): 11–13.

Ultrasound Patterns of Pelvic Masses in Children

Cystic Adnexal Masses

- **Simple ovarian cyst**
- Cystadenoma
- Cystadenofibroma
- Teratoma
- Hydrosalpinx

Complex Adnexal Masses

- Cyst
- **Teratoma**
- Tubo-ovarian abscess
- Dysgerminoma
- **Hemorrhagic cyst**

Solid Adnexal Masses

- Hemorrhagic cyst
- Teratoma
- Dysgerminoma
- Fibroma

Uterine/Vaginal Masses

- Cystic – hydro/hematometrocolpos
- Complex – pregnancy/infection
- Solid – rhabdomyosarcoma, hydatidiform mole

Further Reading

Quillin SP & Siegel MJ (1994) Transabdominal color Doppler ultrasonography of the painful adolescent ovary. *J Ultrasound Med* 13(7): 549–555.

Non-gynecologic Pelvic Masses in Children

Cystic

- **Abscess** – usually secondary to appendicitis
- Lymphocele
- Enteric duplication
- Ureteral dilatation
- Cysts of urachus
- Bladder diverticulum

Complex

- Sacrococcygeal teratoma
- **Abscess**
- Hematoma

Solid

- **Hematoma**
- Neuroblastoma

Congenital Uterine Anomalies

Uterus didelphys	Complete duplication (two uterine horns, two cervices, two vaginas).
Uterus bicornis bicollis	Complete division of uterus down to internal os (one vagina, two cervices, two uterine bodies).
Uterus bicornis unicollis	Partial division of uterus (one vagina, one cervix, two uterine horns).
Uterus unicornis unicollis with a rudimentary remnant	
Septate uterus	Partial or non-resorption of the uterine septum.
Uterus unicornis unicollis	Unilateral arrested development.

11

Fertile and Postmenopausal Women

Non-visualization of Ovary

- Normal ovary obscured by gas – more common on the left side due to sigmoid gas
- Bladder over/underdistended
- Previous oophorectomy
- Displaced – anteversion/retroversion, uterine masses, leiomyoma
- Ectopic ovary – in inguinal canal, failure of descent, low ovary
- Children (commonly seen by modern scanner)
- Postmenopausal – small ovaries
- Atrophic ovaries
- Small ovaries – e.g. Turner's syndrome
- Mullerian dysgenesis
- Distorted pelvic anatomy – previous surgery, previous radiotherapy

Ultrasound Mimics of Ovaries and Ovarian Masses

Low lying cecum	This may mimic an ovarian dermoid. Repeat examination after an enema may reveal its true nature.
Fluid/feces-filled bowel	Demonstrate changes with peristalsis. Reverberation echoes from gas can be mistaken for margins of a mass.
Bladder duplication artifact	This may give rise to pseudomass effect; may be resolved by partial voiding.
Ectopic pregnancy	Usually different clinical setting, e.g. a positive pregnancy test and generally there are no large anechoic spaces.
Hydrosalpinx/pyosalpinx	These may present cystic, solid or complex masses in relation to the adnexa. Hydrosalpinx can become apparent on serial US scanning during ovulation induction by TVS. Hydrosalpinx is usually tubular in shape and often has a folded configuration or short echogenic lines protruding into the lumen.
Vascular aneurysms/ malformations	These show characteristic flow on pulsed Doppler.
Uterine masses	These may present as adnexal masses. Normally ultrasound should be able to differentiate the uterus from the mass. Pedunculated exophytic fibroids are generally solid but there may be a cystic element due to cystic degeneration but usually do not contain large anechoic spaces as do para-ovarian cystadenoma.
Paraovarian cysts	They arise from the mesovarium. Separate from the ovary. Paraovarian cysts with hemorrhage may mimic a cystadenoma; a follow-up US may show resolution.

Paraovarian cystadenoma/ cystadenofibroma	Paraovarian cysts are usually an incidental finding on US and surgery. The majority are simple cysts and diagnosis depends on their paraovarian location quite separate from the ovaries. Cystic masses with solid nodular component are usually ovarian in origin and neoplasm is a strong consideration. Rarely a solid nodular component may be identified within a paraovarian mass. As opposed to paraovarian cysts, which are simple cysts on US, the majority of paraovarian cystadenomas have a nodular component and a minority are septate.
Fallopian tube neoplasms	Fallopian tube neoplasms are rare, generally solid but may have a cystic component and difficult to differentiate from other adnexal masses.
Pelvic kidneys	They have a reniform shape and usually recognizable parenchymal structure. They may become hydronephrotic.
Pseudomyxoma peritonei	This can give rise to a gelatinous material that may implant on serosal surfaces.
Pelvic fat and connective tissue	Any of these structures may be confused with the ovaries. Confusion may be less likely with TVS.
Presacral masses	Their dorsal location may be identified with a water enema technique and computed tomography.
Lymphocele and hematoma	These resemble adnexal cysts and may be difficult to differentiate from gynecologic masses.
Colonic carcinoma	These may present as an 'atypical target sign'. Recurrence after surgery may be difficult to differentiate from other pelvic masses.

Diverticular abscess/ mass	US may reveal bowel wall thickening or fluid surrounding a 'target sign'.
Markedly constipated bowel/rectum	May mimic a dermoid. Rectal examination may identify the cause.
Matted omentum	Polypoid fatty masses which may mimic adnexal tumors. With TVS confusion is less likely.
Obturator internus	May be mistaken for an ovary; this muscle usually lies more posteriorly.
Peritoneal inclusion cysts	In menstruating women with a history of previous pelvic surgery (30–100%). Other causes include trauma, PID and endometriosis. US findings are those of an anechoic septate mass surrounding the ovary. Doppler sonography shows low resistive flow in the septations. The appearance of the ovary inside a large ovoid or irregular fluid collection is characteristic of a peritoneal inclusion cyst.

NB The normal ovary is mobile and may change position.

Further Reading

Kim JS, Lee HJ, Woo SK & Lee TS (1997) Peritoneal inclusion cysts and their relationship to the ovaries: Evaluation with sonography. *Radiology* 204: 481–484.

Kobin CD, Brown DL, Welch WR (1998) Paraovarian cystadenoma and cystadenofibroma: sonographic characteristics in 14 cases. *Radiology* 208: 459–462.

Schiller VL & Tscuchiyama K (1995) Development of hydrosalpinx during ovulation induction. *J Ultra Med* 14: 799–803.

Sohaey R, Gardner TL, Woodward PJ & Peterson M (1995) Sonographic diagnosis of peritoneal inclusion cysts. *J Ultrasound Med* 14: 913–917.

Structures Mistaken for Ovarian Follicles

- Ovarian cyst
- Iliac vessels
- Ovarian vessels
- Uterine vessels
- Hydrosalpinx
- Pyosalpinx

NB The vessels may be mistaken for ovarian follicles in cross-section only. Doppler or color Doppler will differentiate vessels.

Palpable Pelvic Mass Not Seen on Ultrasonography

- No true mass present
- Mass resolved spontaneously
- Mass hidden by bowel loops
- Bowel loops or soft tissues mistaken for mass
- Mass displaced into the abdomen (the position of a mass may vary depending upon the degree of bladder distensions)
- Large ovarian masses may mimic bladder/ascites
- A dermoid or calcified mass giving rise to an echogenic anterior surface with distal shadowing may not give the appearance of a mass (need plain abdominal radiograph) – the 'tip of the iceberg' sign.

Classification of Ovarian Neoplasia

Epithelial tumors (>90% majority benign)

- Serous adenoma and adenocarcinoma
- Mucinous adenoma and adenocarcinoma
- Cystadenofibroma
- Clear cell adenocarcinoma
- Poorly/undifferentiated carcinoma
- Endometroid tumor
- Brenner tumor

Germ cell tumors (make up 30% of ovarian tumors)

- Mature teratoma – benign (dermoid tumor)
- Immature teratoma – malignant
- Dysgerminoma*
- Endodermal sinus tumor*
- Embryonal carcinoma*
- Choriocarcinoma*

Stromal tumors

- Granulosa cell tumor – estrogen producing
- Thecal cell tumor – estrogen producing
- Fibroma
- Luteal cell tumor
- Fibrosarcoma
- Arrhenoblastoma – androgen producing

Ovarian metastases

- Lymphoma
- Leukemia
- GIT – stomach, pancreas, colon
- Bronchus
- Breast

* Malignant tumors.

Bilateral Ovarian Enlargement

- Polycystic ovary syndrome
- Cystic disease
- Ovarian tumors – primary and secondary
- McCune–Albright syndrome
- Hemorrhage

Ovarian Masses

Ovarian cysts

Malignancy is suggested by thick-walled cysts, excrescences, thick septa (especially if incomplete), low pulsatility index <1, resistance index <0.4 (elevated diastolic flow). A unilocular ovarian cyst with a simple cyst appearance and a diameter less than 5 cm is nearly always benign.

(a) **Follicular cysts**

Functional ovarian cysts. Usually small (1–2.5 cm) in diameter, often multiple, thin-walled and occur in an otherwise normal ovary. If these cysts persist they may cause endometrial hyperplasia with associated prominent endometrial echo complex.

(b) **Corpus luteum cysts**

They are usually smooth-walled, anechoic or hypoechoic structures, although they may give the appearances of a complex adnexal mass. Rupture may occur, resulting in free pelvic fluid.

(c) Theca lutein cysts

Often bilateral, thick-walled, well-defined septate structures which may grow to 10 cm in diameter. Theca lutein cysts are usually secondary to an underlying disorder such as hydatidiform mole, choriocarcinoma or ovulation induction therapy.

(d) **Hemorrhagic ovarian cysts**

Both benign and malignant ovarian cysts may be complicated by hemorrhage. The US appearance is very variable, depending on the state of blood within the cyst. The cyst may appear anechoic, solid, complex or septate and debris levels may be present.

(e) **Polycystic ovary**   35–40% – large ovaries with ≥ 5 cysts of 5–8 mm in each ovary, 30% – normal size ovaries. Serial examinations show failure of follicles to change size or configuration. 25% – hypoechoic ovary with no discrete individual cysts, 5% – enlarged ovary isoechoic with uterus. There is a 5–17% risk of ovarian neoplasm and increased incidence of endometrial carcinoma. A normal US does not exclude polycystic ovary syndrome.

(f) Ovarian remnant syndrome   Ovarian remnant syndrome occurs as a result of part of the ovarian tissue being left behind unintentionally after oophorectomy. The remnant may be functional and cystic and produce compression of the distal ureter. This syndrome is considered distinct from residual ovary syndrome, which develops symptoms originating from ovaries preserved at the time of hysterectomy. Ovarian remnant tissue can acquire parasitic blood supply, implant into the peritoneum or other visceral tissue and remains responsive to the hypothalamic–pituitary–ovarian axis. The demonstration of a cystic pelvic mass in a patient with a past history of salpingo-oophorectomy is suggestive of ovarian remnant. Ovarian tissue may get incorporated within a peritoneal cyst. Ovarian remnant syndrome has commonly been described in association with surgery for endometriosis or PID. US: cystic multiseptate mass with a rim of vascularized solid tissue in a patient with a previous history of oophorectomy is highly suggestive of an ovarian remnant syndrome. If a fairly confident diagnosis can be made a US-guided aspiration can be attempted for symptomatic relief.

(g) Paraovarian cysts

These account for 10% of all adnexal masses. They arise from wolffian duct remnants and are usually placed in the broad ligament. They do not regress on serial scans. Hemorrhage, torsion or rupture may occur. A specific diagnosis is not possible unless a normal ovary is identified in addition to an ipsilateral adnexal mass.

(h) **Endometriomas**

Endometriosis is a common condition. (At pelvic surgery 8–20% of women have evidence of endometriosis, presenting as adnexal or pelvic masses.) A more localized form of the disease consists of discrete larger lesions termed endometriomas or 'chocolate cyst'. These are fairly well-defined, thick-walled cysts with low level internal echoes. Recurrent bleeding may give rise to cystic areas with variable internal echoes which may mimic solid masses.

(i) Torsion of the ovary

The risk of torsion increases with ovarian size, particularly with cysts or tumors over 5 cm in diameter. Sonography may reveal a unilaterally enlarged ovary that appears hypoechoic. An associated cystic or solid mass may be seen. Engorged vessels may appear as small multiple cystic structures of uniform size at the periphery of the torted ovary. Associated free fluid may be present in the pelvis in a third of the cases. Identification of the twisted vascular pedicle by US is suggestive of a vascular torsion. CFD can be useful in predicting viability of the twisted adnexal structures by depicting arterial and venous flow.

(j) Hyperstimulated ovary syndrome

Ovarian hyperstimulation may result during assisted conception. It is diagnosed when the ovary measures over 5 cm in the longest diameter and contains multiple follicles. Ascites and pleural effusions can occur. Electrolyte imbalance and venous thrombosis are complications.

(k) **Serous cystadeno-carcinomas**

These neoplasms are quite large, and over half of them are over 15 cm. They are often multi-loculated with thick septa, with numerous papillary projections and echogenic material within the locules.

(l) **Mucinous cystadenomas**

Usually unilateral with prominent septations. The locules may contain low level echoes representing mucin. Rupture of the tumor may cause pseudomyxoma peritonei.

(m) **Serous cystadenoma**

The initial appearance is indistinguishable from a simple cyst. They may be bilateral and can undergo malignant transformation to cystadeno-carcinoma. They are usually unilocular but may contain thin-walled septa with occasionally papillary projections. Ascites may rarely occur.

(n) **Mucinous cystadeno-carcinomas**

These are rare tumors; US features may be indistinguishable from mucinous cystadenomas and serous cystadenocarcinomas. They are bilateral in a quarter of the patients. Metastases from mucinous cystadenocarcinomas or rupture of the tumor may lead to pseudomyxoma peritonei.

(o) **Endometroid carcinoma**

These tumors are frequently bilateral, US appearances are varied and may range from cystic, with papillary projections, to complex solid areas with necrosis and hemorrhage.

(p) Brenner's tumor

See page 382.

(q) **Other cystic masses**

Ectopic pregnancy, pelvic inflammatory disease, pyosalpinx and tubo-ovarian abscesses may be indistinguishable from other adnexal masses on sonography alone. Clinical history is frequently of primary importance in achieving a diagnosis. They may be solid or complex, and are often associated with fluid in the cul-de-sac.

Solid or complex masses

(a) **Endometrial carcinoma**   See page 411.

(b) Clear cell carcinoma   Thought to arise from the Mullerian duct, their US appearances are non-specific and they are usually seen as predominantly solid complex masses.

(c) Brenner's tumor   This is a rare epithelial tumor which is benign and may occur at any age. The turmors are mostly solid, although cystic lesions have been described.

(d) Undifferentiated carcinoma   Usually solid, hypoechoic tumors but may have a complex appearance with areas of cystic necrosis. Prognosis is usually poor.

(e) **Germ cell tumors – teratomas/ dermoids**   These are common tumors in adolescent and young women but may also occur in the elderly. Malignant teratomas are rare. Between 10 and 15 percent of dermoids are bilateral; they often contain fat, teeth and hair and thus have a variable appearance on US. The majority of dermoids are very echogenic and they may shadow. These appearances may be mimicked by bowel or calcified fibroids. Despite the varied appearance of an ovarian teratoma, sonographic features can be distinctive. One such finding is that of a highly echogenic nodule or a 'dermoid plug' within an adnexal mass. A conglomerate of fatty tissue/sebum, hair, teeth and calcification produces the dermoid plug. The size of the dermoid plug varies from a few mm to that occupying the entire mass. Another feature of a teratoma is a highly echogenic focus within the mass due to teeth/calcification that may shadow. Hair may float on top of fatty material – 'tip of iceberg sign'. Fat–fluid level may be seen.

(f) Gonadal stromal tumors

Sex cord-stromal tumors make the largest group of hormone-producing tumors of the ovary but are on the whole uncommon. They include granulosa tumors, fibroma, fibrosarcoma and Sertoli–Leydig tumors. Adult and juvenile types are described while juvenile types occur in children of all ages, adult types usually affect women over the age of 30 years. They are functioning tumors and therefore present early. US: solid; they may be bilateral. Thecoma, fibroma or Brenner's tumor may be associated with Meigs' syndrome, which represents a clinical triad of hydrothorax, benign ascites and an ovarian tumor. Adult granulosa cell tumor may be echogenic but sometimes septate.

(g) Krukenberg's tumors

These represent metastases; 50% are of GIT origin (stomach, colon and pancreas). The most common appearance is of a pelvic mass, usually showing homogeneous low level echoes. Appearances identical to cystadenocarcinoma may occur. Echogenic masses containing variable anechoic spaces have been described.

(h) Lymphoma

Lymphoma of the ovaries is usually a part of more extensive disease and often results from dissemination from other sites. Like lymph nodes, ovarian lymphoma deposits are solid but echo poor. The ovaries are usually enlarged.

(i)	Other ovarian tumors	These include dysgerminoma, choriocarcinoma, embryonal carcinoma and polyembryoma mixed germ cell tumor. Sonographically they are seen as solid or complex masses. Endodermal sinus tumor/yolk sac tumor is the second most common malignant germ cell tumor of the ovary in children accounting for 9–6%. The peak incidence is in the second decade of life. The tumor grows rapidly and symptoms of abdominal pain/palpable abdominal mass are usually of short duration. The tumor secretes α-fetoprotein, which can be used for diagnosis and monitoring. The tumor is aggressive, which had a poor prognosis in the past, however early diagnosis and a combination of surgery and aggressive chemotherapy makes it possible to achieve survival in 80% of patients when the disease is confined to one ovary. US: large complex pelvic mass extending into the abdomen, with both solid and cystic elements, sonography may also show a concurrent dermoid cyst of the ovary, ascites and/or urinary obstruction.
(j)	Solid non-neoplastic masses	Ectopic pregnancy, PID and salpingitis may all present as solid adnexal masses indistinguishable from ovarian masses on sonography alone.

(k) Benign vs malignant ovarian masses

Color flow and pulsed Doppler may help differentiate between malignant lesions and benign lesions; however, there is an overlap between benign and malignant lesions, with inflammatory masses and functioning benign tumors mimicking malignant lesions. Corpus luteum flow cannot be differentiated from flow to malignant lesions. Despite the extensive literature on the subject of benign vs malignant ovarian masses the choices of US features and the role of Doppler remains controversial. Intratumoral blood flow analysis in ovarian cancer does not reveal information on tumor characteristics e.g. staging, histology and morphology of the tumor. However there are 4 sonographic features that as a group are statistically significant features which allow distinction between benign vs malignant masses:

1. The presence and nature of solid component: masses without solid component or markedly hyperechoic solid component are nearly always benign.
2. Presence and location of color Doppler flow: Used only in masses with solid component, pulsed Doppler adds no further distinction.
3. The presence and amount of ascites.
4. The presence and thickness of septations.

Mimics of a 'dermoid plug sign'

- Acute hemorrhage within a pelvic mass – ovarian cyst, endometrioma
- Exophytic lipomatous uterine mass
- Uterus obstructed by endometrial carcinoma
- Perforated appendicitis with an appendolith
- Pyometra/hematometra – elderly
- Ovarian neoplasm with echogenic mural nodules

Unrecognized dermoid plug

- Cystic teratoma confused with bladder
- Bowel gas and fecal material
- May be missed on TVS because of limited field of view
- Rare and revealing feature that may go unrecognized – fat–fluid level
- No true recognition with discovery in a misleading clinical context – teratoma may be an incidental finding

Further Reading

Athey PA, Jayson HT, Estroda R et al (1990) Sonographic findings in primary ovarian pregnancy. *JCU* 18: 730.

Bourne T, Campbell S, Steer C et al (1989) Transvaginal colour flow imaging: a possible new screening technique for ovarian cancer. *BMJ* 299: 1367–1370.

Brown DL, Doubilet PM, Miller FH et al (1998) Benign and malignant ovarian mass: Gray scale and Doppler sonographic features. *Radiology* 208: 103–110.

Crade M (1994) Ovarian cancer: detection by transvaginal ultrasound. A practical approach for clinical practice and review of literature. *Ultrasound Q* 12: 117–126.

Fleischer AC, Roa BK & Kepple DM (1991) Transvaginal color Doppler sonography of ovarian masses. *J Ultrasound Med* 10: 563–565.

Fleischer AC, Tait D, Mayo J et al (1998) Sonographic features of ovarian remnants. *J Ultra Med* 17: 551–552.

Hata K, Hata T (1996) Intratumoral blood flow analysis in ovarian cancer: What does it mean? *J Ultra Med* 15: 571–575.

Ko S-F, Wan Y-L, Ng S-H et al (1999) Adult ovarian granulosa cell tumors: spectrum of sonographic and CT findings with pathologic correlation. *AJR* 172: 1227–1233.

Kurjak A, Aalud I, Alfirevic Z et al (1990) The assessment of abnormal pelvic blood flow by transvaginal color and pulsed Doppler. *Ultrasound Med Biol* 16: 437–442.

Lee EJ, Kwon HC, Hoo HJ et al (1998) Diagnosis of ovarian torsion with color Doppler sonography: Depiction of twisted vascular pedicle. *J Ultra Med* 17: 83–89.

Levintin A, Haller KD, Chen HL et al (1996) Endodermal sinus tumor of the ovary: Imaging evaluation. *AJR* 167: 791–793. Tepper R, Lerner-Geva L, Altaras MM et al (1995) Transvaginal color flow imaging in the diagnosis of ovarian tumors. *J Ultrasound Med* 14: 731–734.

Volpi E, De Grandis T, Zuccaro G et al (1995) Role of transvaginal sonography in the detection of endometrioma. *JCU* 23: 163–167.

Predominantly Solid Adnexal Masses

- Solid teratoma
- **Dermoid cysts**
- GIT metastasis of ovaries
- **Lymphoma of ovaries**
- **Fibroma**
- Arrhenoblastoma
- Granulosa cell tumor

Echogenic Ovarian Tumors

- Adenocarcinoma – without serum or mucous
- Teratoma
- Brenner's tumour
- Fibrothecoma
- Granulosa cell tumor
- Krukenberg's tumor

Ovarian Cancer Risk

- Nulliparity or low parity increases the risk of ovarian cancer; risk decreases with increasing parity
- The use of oral contraceptives is said to associate with low risk
- The risk increases when two or more primary relatives are affected
- The risk increases with advancing age (80% occur over the age of 50 years)
- It takes 2–3 years after menopause for the ovary to atrophy to $2 \times 1.5 \times 0.5$ cm. An ovary larger than this is considered abnormal.
- 80–90% of ovarian cancers have a cystic component
- Even in experienced hands 25–40% of ovaries are not visualized in postmenopausal women both on transabdominal US or TVS
- Benign ovarian cysts occur in 1–14% of postmenopausal women; cysts less than 5 cm in diameter are considered low risk and can be monitored.
- Neither transabdominal US nor TVS have shown acceptable sensitivity or specificity for ovarian cancer screening, although specificity is improved with pelvic examination and tumor marker levels (CA 125)
- CA 125 is a highly non-specific marker with a high degree of overlap between benign and malignant gynecologic disease– a positive CA 125 may bias an ultrasound examination
- CA 125 may be elevated in healthy women (1%), first trimester of pregnancy, cirrhosis, endometriosis and 40% of other intra-abdominal non-ovarian malignancies.
- CA 125 is elevated in only 50% of patients with stage 1 disease, thus half the patients with potentially curable disease will not be detected
- There is considerable overlap of Doppler indices between benign and malignant disease and therefore reliability cannot be placed on these studies. The demonstration of flow on color Doppler in the walls or septae of a cystic ovarian mass does not indicate malignancy

Further Reading

Yamashita Y, Torashima M, Hatanaka Y et al (1995) Adnexal masses: accuracy of characterisation with transvaginal ultrasound and precontrast and postcontrast MR. *Radiology* 194(2): 557–565.

Differential Diagnosis of Cystic Ovarian Masses

- **Follicular cysts**
- Corpus luteum cyst
- Theca luteum cyst
- Polycystic ovary syndrome
- **Endometriosis (chocolate cysts)**
- **Ectopic pregnancy**
- **Tubo-ovarian abscess and PID**
- **Hydrosalpinx**
- Paraovarian cysts
- Hematoma
- Adnexal torsion
- Cystic ovarian tumors
- Peritoneal and mesenteric cysts
- Lymphocele
- Bowel loops
- Bladder diverticulum
- Loculated ascites
- Appendix/diverticula/Crohn's abscess
- Postoperative abscess
- Dermoid
- Degenerated fibroid
- Vascular aneuryms

Adnexal Calcification

- Degenerated tumors (24%)
  Dermoid
  Brenner's tumor
  Adenofibroma ovary
  Thecoma ovary
  Mucinous cystadenoma

- Idiopathic?
  Postulated etiology: previous hemorrhage e.g. cyst, previous infection e.g tubo-ovarian abscess, senescent change related to hormonal environment

- Miscellaneous
  Leiomyoma
  Previous abscess
  Calcified hematoma

NB The shape, size and number of the ovarian calcifications do not seem to be related to the eventual outcome except in one reported patient who had curvilinear calcification, which was eventually found to be related to a mucinous cystadenoma. It has been suggested that the finding of ovarian calcification with otherwise normal US findings warrant some form of follow-up examination.

Focal Calcification in Ovaries

- Calcification in normal ovary – idiopathic – no change over time, laparoscopically normal ovary
- **Dermoid** – punctate calcification
- **Adenofibroma** – multiple punctate calcification
- Mucinous cystadenoma – curvilinear calcification
- Previous tubo-ovarian abscess – punctate calcification
- Previous ovarian torsion

NB   Although calcification in benign tumors tends to be punctate it is possible that curvilinear calcification may be the earliest manifestation of malignancy.

Sonographic Appearance of Endometriosis

Focal disease

- Recurrent bleeding may give rise to cystic areas with variable internal echoes, which may mimic solid masses
- Irregular cystic spaces – chocolate cyst – thick-walled discrete masses with irregular borders and low-level echoes, which may give a solid or complex appearance. These may occur distant to the uterus
- Cysts may contain echogenic material due to blood
- Hypoechoic enlargement of the uterine wall
- Contour anomaly of the uterus
- Thickening of the posterior myometrium may be mistaken for fibroids
- There may be loss of definition of pelvic organs

Diffuse disease

- The scans may appear normal, as the lesions are small and scattered and not detectable
- Multiple cysts may be detectable bilaterally

Differential Diagnosis of Endometriosis

- Uterine fibroids
- Nabothian cysts – small fluid-filled spaces in the myometrium near the cervix due to retention cysts of cervical glands
- Cystic or solid ovarian tumors
- Uterine tumors
- Tubo-ovarian abscess
- PID
- Ectopic pregnancy
- Hemorrhagic cyst

Endometrial Thickness

A thickened endometrium is a sensitive but non-specific indicator of endometrial disease; it is used as a screening tool by most gynecologists. Dilatation and curettage is unguided and not an exact tool as focal masses and skip lesions of the endometrium may be missed. Only 60% of the endometrial surface is actually sampled at D&C. Hysteroscopy is sensitive but invasive. There is considerable disagreement in the literature about normal endometrial thickness but 4 mm or less even in women with bleeding is associated with endometrial atrophy. For women who are asymptomatic a threshold of 8–10 mm is suggested. Baldwin et al using hysterosonography and TVS have recognized a specific sign for a focal endometrial process. This sign consists of a hyperechoic line, partially or completely surrounding a central echo-complex. This line can be seen with many intracavitary processes including polyps, submucosal fibroids, foci of asymmetric hyperplasia and localized neoplasia. All these processes are best managed with hysteroscopy.

- Diffuse process – no hyperechoic line
- Focal process – hyperechoic line

Increased Endometrial Thickness

- **Early intrauterine pregnancy (decidual reaction)**
- **Hormonal excess – endogenous/exogenous**
- **Decidual reaction with ectopic pregnancy**
- **Retained products of conception**
- Anovulatory cycles
- **Gestational trophoblastic disease**
- **Endometrial carcinoma** (postmenopausal women with endometrial thickness greater than 4 mm requires histology or monitoring)
- **Endometrial polyp**
- Hematometra
- **Tamoxifen therapy**
- Pyometra
- Cervical pregnancy
- Adenomyosis
- Endometrial hyperplasia
- Hormone replacement therapy: HRT has greater endometrial thickness than controls and show most variation in measurements. They should undergo US either early or late in the hormone cycle to evaluate the endometrium at its thinnest

- Idoxifen is a selective estrogen receptor that has beneficial effects on bone turnover. The drug is associated with a dose-related increase in endometrial thickness and endometrial fluid as assessed by TVS but not associated with estrogenic effect on endometrial histologic features
- Asymptomatic treated hypertensive patients as compared to normotensive or untreated hypertensives – average endometrial thickness: calcium-channel blockers: 5.4 mm, ACE inhibitors: 6.5 mm, β-adrenergic antagonists: 6.9 mm
- Endometrial malacoplakia

Polypoid Echogenic Endometrial Mass

- Endometrial carcinoma
- Endometrial hyperplasia
- Pyometra
- Hydatiform mole
- Incomplete abortion
- Submucosal fibroids – usually hypoechoic
- Mixed mesodermal tumor
- Uterine sex cord-stromal tumor: rare endometrial tumor resembling ovarian sex cord-stromal tumors, clinically benign unless they rupture, are very large or associated with severe cytologic atypia, mimic endometrial polyp on US.

Further Reading

Alcazar JL (2000) Endometrial sonographic findings in asymptomatic hypertensive postmenopausal women. *JCU* 28: 175–178.

Bader-Armstrong B, Shah Y & Rubens D (1989) Use of ultrasound and magnetic resonance imaging in the diagnosis of cervical pregnancy. *JCU* 17: 283.

Baldwin MT, Dudiak KM, Gorman B & Marks CA (1999) Focal intracavitary masses recognised with the hyperechoic line sign of endovaginal US and characterized with hysterosonography. *Radiographics* 19: 927–935.

Brandt KR, Thurmond AS & McCarthy JL (1996) Focal calcifications in an otherwise normal ovaries. *Radiology* 198: 415–417.

Bree RL, Bowerman RA, Bohm-Valez M et al (2000) US evaluation of the uterus in patients with postmenopausal bleeding: A positive effect on diagnostic decision making. *Radiology* 216: 260–264.

Fleischer AC, Wheeler JE, Yeh I-T et al (1999) Sonographic assessment of the endometrium in osteopenic postmenopausal women treated with idoxifen. *J Ultra Med* 18: 503–512.

Franco A, Aquino NM, Malik SL & Navarro C (1999) Sonographic presentation of uterine sex cord-stromal tumor. *JCU* 27: 199–201.

Granberg S, Wikland M, Karlsson N et al (1991) Endometrial thickness as measured by endovaginal ultrasonography for identifying endometrial abnormality. *Am J Obstet Gynecol* 164: 47–52.

Levine D, Gosink BB & Johnson LA (1995) Changes in endometrial thickness in postmenopausal women undergoing hormone replacement therapy. *Radiology* 97: 603–608.

Lin MC, Gosink BB, Wolf SI et al (1991) Endometrial thickness after menopause: effect of hormonal replacement. *Radiology* 180: 427–432.

Malpini A, Singer J, Wolverson MK & Merenda G (1990) Endometrial hyperplasia: value of endometrial thickness in ultrasonographic diagnosis and clinical significance. *JCU* 18: 173–177.

Riccio GJ, Jorizzo JR, Chen MYM (2000) Sonohysterographic findings of endometrial malacoplakia. *J Ultra Med* 19: 415–417.

Thurmond AS (1995) Ultrasound of infertility and uterine anomalies. *Ultrasound Q* 13: 87–102.

Varner RE, Sparks JM, Cameron CD et al (1991) Transvaginal sonography of the endometrium in post-menopausal women. *Obstet Gynecol* 78: 195–199.

Classification of Gestational Trophoblastic Disease

Gestational trophoblastic disease

Gestational trophoblastic disease is a neoplastic disorder of the trophoblast that may present in a relatively benign form – hydatidiform mole or more malignant forms such as an invasive mole or choriocarcinoma. Classified as complete moles, which consist of trophoblastic tissue only or incomplete moles that contain both trophoblastic tissue and fetal parts. The trophoblastic tissue show an abnormal chromosomal karyotype and is associated with raised levels of hCG. They represent less than 1% of all gynecological malignancies. Risk factors include maternal age >35 or <20 years of age, previous molar pregnancy and previous spontaneous abortions.

Complete mole

Hydatidiform mole/molar pregnancy/complete mole/classic mole. Presents clinically as uterus too large for dates, severe pre-eclampsia before 24 weeks gestation, first-trimester vaginal bleeding, and passage of grape-like vesicles per vagina. Rarely hyperthyroidism may occur due to production of TSH activity by the trophoblast. Echogenic material fills the uterus, there is no fetal tissue, the mass is echogenic but does not cause a great deal of ultrasound beam attenuation. Vesicles are usually less than 1.5 cm in the first trimester but may be over 2 cm in diameter in the second trimester. Later confluent hypoechoic areas occur due to hemorrhage. Ovarian cysts may be evident (30–50%).

Complete mole with coexistent fetus

This is a rare occurrence and is usually due to molar degeneration of a dizygotic twin. The hCG is markedly elevated and is not explainable on a normal pregnancy. Patients present with vaginal bleeding in the second trimester and a large-for-dates uterus. Amniocentesis reveals a normal karyotype thus eliminating a partial mole. US shows a normal fetus and placenta associated with echogenic material – representing the hydatidiform mole. Ovarian cysts may be apparent. Unlike partial moles these demonstrate the same potential for malignant change as the classical moles and may be due to a twin pregnancy, one fertilized product giving rise to the mole.

Partial mole

Coexistent mole and fetal parts. The fetus shows multiple anomalies and severe IUGR. There is a high incidence of chromosomal abnormalities in the fetus. Sonographic demonstration of molar vesicles together with a well-formed fetus and a normal placenta suggest coexistent moles and fetus.

Invasive mole

Locally invasive hydatidiform mole accounts for up to 15% of cases sonographically. There is often (75%) a history of previous molar pregnancy. Seen as an enlarged uterus containing a molar mass with foci of increased echogenicity extending into the myometrium. Anechoic areas of hemorrhage and necrosis and appearances may be indistinguishable from other uterine tumors. Large ovarian cysts may be apparent.

Hydropic degeneration of placenta

Hydropic degeneration is not a hydatidiform mole variant because it involves the placenta without histologic evidence of trophoblastic proliferation. The overall appearances depend upon the extent of vesicular change, hemorrhage, necrosis and breakdown products of conception. It may be very difficult to differentiate from a partial mole sonographically.

Choriocarcinoma

Choriocarcinoma is the most malignant form of trophoblastic disease. Nearly half the cases are preceded by molar pregnancy, whilst only 3–5% of molar pregnancies are complicated by a choriocarcinoma. Choriocarcinoma is also associated with spontaneous abortion (25%), normal pregnancy (22%) and ectopic pregnancy (2.5%). Clinically they present with continued vaginal bleeding and a continued elevation of hCG after expulsion of a molar pregnancy or normal delivery. Choriocarcinoma metastasize to the liver, lung, brain, bone and the GIT. US: echogenic mass enlarging the uterus surrounding by irregular sonolucent areas due to hemorrhage/necrosis. Liver metastases may be detected sonographically. Theca lutein cysts are seen frequently.

Placental site trophoblastic tumor

This is rare neoplasm, considered by some to be variant of choriocarcinoma. The tumor arises from intermediate trophoblast cells within the placental bed. In the majority of patients the tumor runs a benign course, however disseminated disease may be fatal. The levels of hCG are low as compared to gestational trophoblastic disease. The tumor can be distinguished from a hydatidiform mole by the absence of chorionic villi and from a choriocarcinoma by the absence of necrosis and hemorrhage. The US appearances may mimic an invasive mole.

Pelvic Masses During Pregnancy

Physiologic Masses

Corpus luteum cyst	The cysts may at times exceed 10 cm (usually <3 cm). Adnexal cysts in the first trimester are regarded as luteal cysts and observed.
Bowel loop	Bowel loop/pelvic cecum may mimic adnexal mass.
Pelvic kidney	

Pathologic Masses

Endometriomas	These represent ectopic endometrial tissue and have been reported in a variety of organs. The most common form presents as tiny pelvic deposits not visible on ultrasound. Sonography identifies endometrial tissue presenting as adnexal or pelvic mass lesions. Termed 'chocolate cysts', they present as fairly well-defined masses with thick walls. Low-level echoes and/or fluid debris levels can be identified. Highly reflective echoes within the mass may represent recent hemorrhage. Endometriomas may at times be purely cystic.
Ovarian neoplastic cysts	These include cystadenomas, cystic teratomas and cystadenocarcinomas (exceedingly rare in pregnancy). Ultrasound is usually unable to differentiate between benign and malignant lesions, although transvaginal duplex sonography has the potential for distinguishing between benign and malignant ovarian tumors based on detection of low resistance flow.

Myomas	Usually hypoechoic, may attenuate the ultrasonic beam; their mass effect may distort the contour of the uterus. Occasional myomas are heterogeneous. Myomas may cause obstructed delivery and/or fetal malposition, therefore position and size are important. May undergo rapid growth and central necrosis – seen as a tender, mixed echogenic mass.
Solid ovarian tumors	These include teratomas, carcinomas and lymphomas. While lymphomas are usually echo poor, the other tumors are of varying echogenicity.
Non-neoplastic adnexal tumors	These include pedunculated leiomyomas and ovarian pregnancy.
Abscess	These may be tubo-ovarian, appendiceal or Crohn's abscesses.
Miscellaneous cystic masses	Mesenteric, enteric, urachal, echinococcal, peritoneal inclusion cysts, lymphoceles and hydrosalpinx also appear cystic.
Neurogenic masses	Schwannomas.

Further Reading

Athey PA, Jayson HT, Estroda R et al (1990) Sonographic findings in primary ovarian pregnancy. *JCU* 18: 730.

Bourne T, Campbell S, Steer C et al (1989) Transvaginal colon flow imaging. A possible new screening technique for ovarian cancer. *BMJ* 299: 1367–1370.

Callen PW (ed.) (1994) *Ultrasonography in Obstetrics and Gynecology*, 3rd edn, pp 82–83. Philadelphia: WB Saunders.

Fleischer AC, Rao BK & Keepple DM (1991) Transvaginal color Doppler sonography of ovarian masses. *J Ultrasound Med* 10: 563–565.

Kurjak A, Aalud I, Alfirevic Z et al (1990) The assessment of abnormal pelvic blood flow by transvaginal color and pulsed Doppler. *Ultrasound Med Biol* 16: 437–422.

Prominent Endometrial Echo Complex

Decidual reaction

Decidual reaction secondary to hormonal stimulation of the endometrium is normally present in intrauterine pregnancy. Decidual reaction is represented sonographically by echogenic, thickened endometrium. Decidual reaction may occur in 20-50% of ectopic pregnancies.

Secretory phase of menstrual cycle

Sonography demonstrates cyclical changes in the normal endometrium. The endometrium becomes thickened and echogenic in the secretory phase.

Stimulated endometrium

The endometrium in postmenopausal women is usually thin, no more than 4 mm. Hormonal stimulation by medications such as estrogens for osteoporosis may alter the thickness and echogenicity of the endometrium.

Endometrial carcinoma

See page 411.

Endometrial hyperplasia

This is related to proliferation of glands and stroma caused by prolonged and persistent estrogenic stimulation, and is the most common cause of uterine bleeding. It can occur during menstrual years as well as in the post-menopausal years. Classified pathologically into simple, complex and atypical hyperplasia, the incidence of subsequent malignancy is as high as 25-50% in the atypical variety.

Endometritis

Bacterial infection of the endometrium may occur postpartum, following abortion or due to the presence of an IUCD. The uterus may appear normal or may be enlarged, with a wide echogenic cavity which may contain air or fluid.

Endometrial polyp   See page 411.

Pendunculated   See page 410.
endometrial leiomyomas

Retained products of   The appearances of the 'endometrial complex'
conception   depend upon the stage of the pregnancy at
                           which abortion occurred and the tissue type of
                           the retained product, e.g. osseous.

Persistent corpus   These cysts elaborate progesterone, which is
luteum cysts   likely to sustain secretory endometrium.

IUCD with progesterone   The combination gives rise to an echogenic and
                           thickened endometrium.

Hematometra   This has several causes. The presence of
                           blood within the endometrial cavity alters its
                           echogenicity, depending on the stage of
                           resolution of the blood/clot.

Malignant mixed   In common with other uterine tumors,
Mullerian tumor   particularly those involving the endometrium,
                           malignant mixed Mullerian tumors may enhance
                           the endometrial echoes.

Cervical pregnancy   The sonographic criteria for cervical pregnancy
                           are: uterine enlargement, diffuse echogenic
                           intrauterine echoes, enlarged cervix and absent
                           intrauterine pregnancy.

Gestational trophoblastic See page 398.
disease

Adenomyosis   Characteristically cause uterine and contour
enlargement   anomaly with a normal central echo, although
                           on rare occasions the endometrial echo com-
                           plex may be prominent.

Tamoxifen therapy

Tamoxifen is widely used in the treatment of carcinoma of the breast. US abnormalities of the uterine endometrium have been observed in these patients

1. endometrial thickness >4 mm;
2. endometrium may be hypoechoic, homogeneous or hyperechoic with multiple small cystic spaces;
3. endometrial polyps with cyst within them;
4. endometrial carcinoma.

Further Reading

Bader-Armstrong B, Shah Y & Rubens D (1989) Use of ultrasound and magnetic resonance imaging in the diagnosis of cervical pregnancy. *JCU* 17: 283.

Faustin D, Chan PC & Pase M (1987) Intrauterine pregnancy following conservative treatment of cervical pregnancy. *J Ultrasound Med* 6: 467–470.

Forrest TS, Elyaderane MK, Mullenberg RI et al (1988) Cyclical endometrial changes. US assessment with histologic correlation. *Radiology* 167: 233.

Hulka CA & Hall DA (1993) Endometrial abnormalities associated with tamoxifen therapy for breast carcinoma. *AJR* 160: 809–812.

Lin MC, Gosink BB, Wolf SI et al (1991) Endometrial thickness after menopause: effect of hormonal replacement. *Radiology* 180: 427–432.

Malpini A, Singer J, Wolverson MK et al (1990) Endometrial hyperplasia: value of endometrial thickness in ultrasonographic diagnosis and clinical significances. *JCU* 18: 173–177.

Stadtmauer L & Grunfeld L (1995) The significance of endometrial filling defects detected on routine transvaginal sonography. *J Ultrasound Med* 14: 169–172.

Varner RE, Sparks JM, Cameron CD et al (1991) Transvaginal sonography of the endometrium in post-menopausal women. *Obstet Gynecol* 78: 195–199.

Woman I, Sagi J, Ginat S et al (1996) The sensitivity and specificity of vaginal sonography in detecting endometrial abnormalities in women with post-menopausal bleeding. *JCU* 24: 79–82.

Endometrial Fluid Collection

Physiologic

- At the time of menses
- Normal gestation sac
- Decidual reaction in contralateral bicornuate horn
- In the neonatal period in response to maternal hormonal stimulation in utero

Complicated pregnancy

- Blighted ovum and missed abortion
- Pseudogestational sac of ectopic pregnancy
- Incomplete abortion
- Retained products of conception

Inflammation/infection

- Endometriosis
- Salpingitis
- PID

Hemorrhage

- Normal/dysfunctional
- After dilatation and curettage
- Ruptured corpus luteum cyst

Neoplasia

- Cervical carcinoma
- Adenomyosis
- Degenerating fibroids
- Hydatidiform mole
- Choriocarcinoma
- Uterine sarcoma
- Benign cystic teratoma

Genital tract occlusion

- (Causing hydrometra, hematometra or pyometra)
- Cervical obstruction, whatever the cause
- Cervical stenosis
- Cervical carcinoma
- Endometrial carcinoma
- Imperforate hymen
- Previous cervical surgery

Iatrogenic/traumatic

- After dilatation and curettage
- Uterine perforation
- Drainage of free peritoneal fluid via genital tract

NB Endometrial fluid collections found in asymptomatic postmenopausal women still may be associated with endometrial malignancy even in the presence of thin endometrium.

Further Reading

Cunate JS, Dunne MG & Butler M (1984) Sonographic diagnoses of uterus perforation following suction curettage. *JCU* 1: 108.

Lister JE, Kane GJ, Ehrmann RL et al (1988) Ultrasound appearances of adenomyosis mimicking adenocarcinoma in post-menopausal women. *JCU* 16: 519.

Zalel Y, Tepper R, Chen I et al (1996) Clinical significance of endometrial fluid collections in asymptomatic postmenopausal women. *J Ultra Med* 15: 513–515.

Echogenic Foci within the Uterine Cavity

Intrauterine contraceptive devices

High-amplitude echoes in the uterine cavity which remain at low gain setting with entrance and exit echoes giving a parallel line appearance are seen in 65% of cases, ± distal acousting shadowing. Configuration of the echoes reflect the type of IUCD. Women with an IUCD in situ who become pregnant are at increased risk of ectopic pregnancy.

Calcifications

Commonly associated with myomas, which may appear intrauterine with the submucous variety.

Retained products of conception

Bright echoes may be demonstrated within the uterus, particularly if osseous parts are retained.

Radiation therapy implants

These may cause high-intensity echoes within the uterine cavity which may shadow. History of implant insertion may be obtained.

Air within the uterine cavity

This usually follows dilatation and curettage or culdiocentesis.

Cerclage sutures

They may mimic IUCDs; an obvious history may be obtained.

Intrauterine osseous metaplasia (osteoid tissue)

This may be the result of previous pregnancy or inflammation.

Further Reading

Roberts CE & Athey PA (1992) Sonographic demonstration of air in the myometrium. A complication of culdiocentesis. *J Ultrasound Med* 11: 7–9.

Effects of Exposure to Diethylstilbestrol

- Increased incidence of vaginal carcinoma
- Increased incidence of genital anomalies

Abnormal vaginal mucosa	56%
Vaginal adenosis	33%
Vaginal fibrous ridges	22%
Small T-shaped uterus	

Uterine Neoplasms/Masses

Leiomyomas (fibroids)   Common smooth muscle tumors, found in 20% of women >35 years. They are more common in Afro-Caribbeans. Leiomyomas exhibit a variety of US appearances. The tumors may be hyperechoic or hypoechoic, homogeneous or heterogeneous, sound-enhancing or sound-attenuating attributed to tissue component and areas of degeneration within the tumors primarily of smooth muscle tend to be hypoechoic and homogeneous but become increasingly heterogeneous and echogenic when complicated by hemorrhage, necrosis, fibrosis and calcification. They often cause acoustic shadowing – discrete shadows not arising from echogenic foci but result from structural features of the leiomyomas at the transitional boundaries between juxtaposed tissue types or at the curved margins of organized anatomic structures. Sonographic estimates of size, number and position are frequently impossible when discrete masses cannot be discerned. Several secondary US signs can indicate their presence: enlarged but normally shaped uterus, an indentation on the contour of the urinary bladder, subtle hetero-geneous echo texture of myometrium or an irregular lobular contour of the uterus, sub-stantial acoustic attenuation or shadowing. The presence of shadowing and acoustic attenu-ation is virtually a defining characteristic of leiomyomas.

Endometrial carcinoma

Over 70% occur at >50 years, with peak incidence at age 62. Sonographic diagnosis remains difficult because early lesions may be confined to the corpus (stage I) or extend into the cervix (stage II) and may not alter the uterine echo pattern. The presence of prominent endometrial echo complex >4 mm in a woman with post-menopausal bleeding and irregularity or loss of the normal endometrial/myometrial junction is suggestive of this diagnosis. Endometrial carcinomas may obstruct the uterine cavity causing hydrometra, pyometra or hematometra. A fluid/debris level may be identified. Occasionally, spread to other organs in the pelvis may be identified on US. Low-impedance flow is observed in various diseases of the endometrium, with an overlap between pulsatility index (PI) and resistive index (RI) of benign and malignant lesions. Endometrial thickness <6–8 mm usually excludes the diagnosis of endometrial carcinoma.

Endometrial polyp

May occur in all ages, but are more common at menopause. Sonography may reveal discrete mass(es) within the uterine cavity, enlargement of the uterus and prominent endometrial echo complex.

Adenomyosis

Common gynecological disorder that affects women of reproductive age with a reported incidence in unselected hysterectomy specimens range from 8.8% to 31%. Until recently the diagnosis was rarely established before hysterectomy. Invasion by nests of endometrial tissue causes uterine enlargement. The presenting symptoms of pelvic pain, dysmenorrhea and menorrhagia are non-specific and may occur with other gynecologic disorders. The rate of pre-operative diagnosis on clinical grounds is poor at 2.6–26%. Recent studies with MRI and US have improved diagnosis. The myometrial echo pattern, central echo complex and uterine contour may be normal. Occasionally, adenomyosis is focal, which may result in contour abnormality, although the central echo complex is normal. Rarely a honeycomb appearance caused by cystic spaces is encountered. Pelvis endometriosis and adenomyosis may coexist in 30% of patients. US: hypoechoic/heterogeneous with cysts – 40%, hypoechoic/heterogeneous areas – 44%, hypoechoic areas with cysts – 12%, and heterogeneous areas – 4%. Mottled heterogeneous myometrium, a globular asymmetric uterus, small myometrial lucent areas with indistinct endometrial stripe is said to be suggestive of adenomyosis.

Cervical carcinoma

Sonographically there may be a solid retrovesical mass indistinguishable from a cervical leiomyoma. Clinical and magnetic resonance staging are more accurate than US. Intracervical US with a high-frequency miniature probe: accurate staging in patients with early stage cancer is crucial in determining the most appropriate treatment. TVS, CT and MR imaging are currently the imaging of choice in staging of invasive cervical cancer. However these techniques cannot diagnose microinvasion. Intracervical US has been recently used and found useful in early invasion. TVS and TRUS are said to be as accurate as MR and more accurate than CT in staging cervical cancer. However all these techniques have limitation of image resolution making detection of early cancer difficult. Because high-frequency probes theoretically have resolution of <1 mm, some micro-invasion is expected to be detectable. The use of intracavitary MR techniques may surmount the limitation of resolution.

Uterine sarcoma

Rare tumors (3% of all uterine tumors). All age groups are affected, but the majority are approximately 60 years. Leiomyosarcomas are believed to arise from pre-existing leiomyomas. Uterine sarcomas may be indistinguishable from large leiomyomas. Commonly, large tumors present with areas of hemorrhage and/or necrosis, with bizarre areas of high-intensity echoes, invasion into the other pelvic organs may be seen as an extrauterine mass. Metastases to the liver suggest leiomyosarcoma. A malignant mixed Mullerian tumor often presents as a bulky uterus with polypoid tumors filling the endometrial cavity and protruding from the cervical os.

Uterine AVM

Uterine arteriovenous malformations are rare and can be classified into congenital and acquired forms. The congenital types are related to anomalous differentiation in the primitive capillary plexus, which results in an abnormal communication between arteries and veins. Histologically they appear as multiple cirsoid or cavernous on the basis of the diameter of the intratumoral vessels in an otherwise healthy woman with no hemodynamic effects. The acquired type of AVM are more common and usually traumatic: spontaneous abortions, D&C, therapeutic abortion, endometrial carcinoma, gestational trophoblastic disease, cesarian secti and DES exposure. Symptoms may be acute or chronic: menorrhagia or menometrorrhagia, which requires blood transfusion in 30% of reported cases. US: Gray scale rarely performed, a conventional TVS may also be confusing but application of color/conventional Doppler allows correct identification.

Further Reading

Bromley B, Shipp TD, Benacerraf B (2000) Adenomyosis: sonographic findings and diagnostic accuracy. *J Ultra Med* 19: 529–534.

Cobby M, Browning J, Jones A et al (1990) Magnetic resonance imaging, computed tomography and endosonography in local staging of carcinoma of the cervix. *Br J Radiol* 63: 673–679.

Huang MW, Muradali D, Thurston WA, Wilson SR (1998) Uterine arteriovenous malformation: Gray-scale and Doppler US features with MR correlation. *Radiology* 206: 115–123.

Kikuchi A, Okai T, Kobayashi K et al (1996) Intracervical US with high frequency miniature probe: A method of diagnosing early invasive cervical cancer. *Radiology* 198: 411–413.

Kliewer MA, Hertzberg BS, George PY et al (1995) Acoustic shadowing from uterine leiomyomas: sonographic-pathologic correlation. *Radiology* 196: 99–102.

Reinhold C, Atri M, Mehio A et al (1995) Diffuse uterine adenomyosis: morphologic criteria and diagnostic accuracy of endo-vaginal sonography. *Radiology* 197: 609–614.

Sheth S, Hamper UM, McCollum ME et al (1995) Endometrial blood flow analysis in postmenopausal women: can it help differentiate benign from malignant causes of endometrial thickening. *Radiology* 195: 661–665.

Yacoe ME & Brooke J (1995) Degenerated uterine leiomyoma mimicking acute appendicitis: sonographic diagnoses. *JCU* 23: 473–475.

Uterine Lipomatous Tumors

These tumors are rare with an incidence of 0.005–0.2%. The clinical presentation is similar to leiomyomas, including uterine enlargement, chronic pelvic discomfort, heaviness and bleeding. US: lipomatous tumors can be diagnosed with a high degree of certainty by transabdominal or TVS by features of a fairly well-defined, homogeneous hyperechoic uterine mass with shadowing. Lipomatous uterine tumors:

- Pure lipoma
- Lipoleiomyoma
- Fibromyolipoma
- Myolipoma

Further Reading

Serafini G, Martinoli C, Quadri P et al (1996) Lipomatous tumors of the uterus: ultrasonographic findings in 11 cases. *J Ultra Med* 16: 195–199.

Fluid in the Cul-de-Sac

Blood	Normal ovulation, ruptured ovarian cyst, ruptured ectopic pregnancy, endometriosis, trauma and postoperative.
Transudate	Part of generalized ascites, e.g. heart failure.
Exudate	Pelvic inflammatory disease, part of generalized exudative ascites, e.g. malignancy.
Encapsulated collections	Bowel, ovarian cyst, endometrioma, abscess, urinoma and lymphocele.

Further Reading

Schellpfeffer MA (1995) Sonographic detection of free pelvic fluid. *J Ultrasound Med* 14: 205-209.

Differential Diagnosis of Vaginal Masses

Cystic Masses

Hematocolpos

Obstruction of the genital canal may occur from several causes, and may result in the collection of blood (hematometra), fluid (hydrometra) or pus (pyometra) in the uterus. Sonographically, there is a cystic distention of the genital canal; the size and location of the fluid collection depend upon the site of obstruction. Hematocolpos is the collection of blood within the vagina.

Gartner's duct cyst

These usually lie proximal to the vagina in the adnexa or along the anterolateral aspect of the vaginal wall. Arising from mesonephric duct remnants, they are the most common cystic vaginal masses. They are usually incidental findings.

Vaginal inclusion cysts

These are related to the inclusion of the vaginal epithelium during surgery and usually found as cystic masses in the posterior or lateral wall of the vagina.

Mucinous cysts

These are related to a developmental anomaly due to remnants of the incomplete separation of the rectum and urogenital sinus by the urachal fold.

Endometriosis

Aberrant endometrial tissue may be present in the vagina, the most common site being the posterior fornix. It may be entirely cystic, or may appear as a complex mass. The mass may be subject to cyclical change.

Urethral diverticula	Usually acquired, they are said to be present in 3% of asymptomatic women, but are an often overlooked cause of lower urinary tract symptoms. They may occur anywhere along the urethra but most are found in the midurethra. The size may vary from millimeters to several centimeters and may be multilocular. Calculi and/or tumors may occur within the diverticula.
Ureteroceles	In about 40% of ureteroceles, the orifice opens outside the bladder, proximal or distal to the external sphincter. These cystic swellings may project into the vagina and can be recognized on sonography.
Cystoceles	This is a form of vaginal prolapse of the bladder and urethra. Sonography may reveal a midline cystic swelling in the vagina in communication with the bladder.
Bartholin gland abscess	Bartholin glands are paired vulvovaginal mucus-secreting epithelial lined glands. These glands drain via ducts (approximately 2.5 cm) at the junction of hymen and labia minora at the posterolateral aspect of the vagina. Lined by transitional epithelium these ducts are particularly prone to obstruction at their ostia. Accumulation of secretions within these ducts give rise to cystic dilatation, which may get inflamed and infected. Treatment is surgical. This is particularly the case over the age of 40 years because of the risk of a Bartholin gland carcinoma. Sonography reveals a hypoechoic mass with a small anechoic component concentrically surrounded by multiple echogenic layers. On transperineal sonography a cystic structure is seen in relation to the bulbous urethra with septations or internal echoes. Ultrasound would rule out lesions such as urethral tumors.

Solid Masses

Foreign body	Foreign body, e.g. tampon (appearance is variable) may be seen as a very echogenic mass with shadowing, but when soaked in fluid the texture of the material may be discernible on US. The possibility of a foreign body should always be remembered in children, who may give no history of insertion of the article, which may have been present for some time.
Leiomyoma	Pedunculated leiomyomas may prolapse through the cervix into the vagina and be seen as a hypoechoic mass.
Leiomyoma of the urethra	This has been described as a well-defined, hypoechoic mass in the region of the urethra, in relationship to the anterior vagina/vulva on transvaginal sonography.
Vaginal polyp	They may be single or multiple finger-like projections; either echogenic or low reflectivity on US.
Neoplasms	True vaginal tumors are rare in children and uncommon in adults. Clear cell carcinoma may be associated with DES exposure in utero. Primary and secondary tumors are usually seen as solid heterogeneous masses.

Vaginal Malignant Neoplasms

- Carcinoma in situ
- Invasive epidermoid carcinoma
- Adenocarcinoma (age group 7–29 years)
- Melanoma
- Fibrosarcoma
- Leiomyosarcoma
- Sarcoma botryoides (girls under 5 years)
- Endodermal sinus tumor
- Metastatic carcinoma
  Choriocarcinoma
  Cervix
  Endometrium
  Bladder
  Rectum

Female Urethra

Urethral sphincter

The female urethral sphincter (the external rhabdosphincter of the bladder) is regularly observed on routine scanning of the female bladder. This sphincter which has been dubbed as the 'female pseudoprostate', is seen as a rounded or oval midline structure, which measures 1.30 cm × 1.33 cm × 0.96 cm in longitudinal, transverse and antero-posterior dimensions at the bladder base. The structure is fairly well defined and rounded. This is a normal anatomical structure and should not be confused with a pathological polyp/mass.

Acquired urethral diverticula

These occur in 3% of asymptomatic women. However they may be an overlooked cause of persistent urinary symptoms on the face of normal routine urological investigations. Symptoms are often mistaken for cystitis, stress incontinence, infected periurethral glands or endometriosis. The standard technique for investigating suspected urethral diverticula is retrograde urethrography or voiding cystourethrography. Sonography is useful in women with suspected urethral diverticula. Several approaches have been used including perineal, transrectal, TVS and transurethral sonography. Endoscopic urethral US appears particularly good and provides information on the extent and location of the diverticular neck, both important in surgical excision. The technique also provides information on lesions connected to the urethra. The diverticula appear as echopoor masses with a debris level.

Differential Diagnosis of Female Urethral Diverticula

- Urethral diverticula
- Gartner's duct cysts
- Endometriosis
- Ectopic ureteroceles
- Vaginal inclusion cysts
- Skene gland abscesses
- Hematoma
- Accessory phallic urethra with obstructed and dilated dorsal urethra

Urethral Tumors in a Female

Benign

- Polyp*
- Papilloma*
- Adenoma*

Malignant

- Transitional cell carcinoma (proximal urethra)
- Squamous cell carcinoma (distal urethra)

Further Reading

Lorion JL, Paula CC, Wacquez M & Connay M (1992) Leiomyoma of the urethra: appearances on transvaginal sonography. *AJR* 158: 694.

Rasines GL, Gutierrez MR, Abascal FA & De Diego AC (1996) Female urethral diverticula: value of transrectal sonography. *JCU* 24: 90–92.

Sanders R, Genadry R, Yarg A & Mostwin J (1994) Imaging of the female urethra with ultrasound. *Ultrasound Q* 12: 167–183.

* Recorded association with malignancy.

12

Obstetric and Gynecologic Emergencies and Non-obstetric Emergencies Peculiar to Pregnancy

Obstetric

Ectopic pregnancy

See page 371.

Cervical incompetence

Common cause of pregnancy failure in the second trimester, which may present with premature rupture of membrane resulting in OH. US: bulging of fetal membranes into a widened internal os and shortening of the cervical canal, TVS is more accurate. Normal mean cervical length is 3 cm, but because of dynamic nature of cervical canal during pregnancy, the normal length of a competent cervix falls within a wide range. Determination of closed length of the cervix may be used as a prognostic risk factor for the risk of preterm labour.

Retroplacental hematoma abruptio and placentae

Hemorrhage along the basal plate, separating the placenta from the uterine wall may result from rupture of spiral arteries due to maternal hypertension, trauma, smoking, acute chorioamnioitis, alcohol and cocaine abuse and retroplacental myomas. US: retroplacental may mimic a thickened placenta, which may be hypoechoic or heterogeneous and because US may not be able to detect small retroplacental hematoma, a negative scan does not rule out the presence of placental abruption.

Uterine dehiscence and rupture

Rupture may occur in a normal uterus but old cesarean scars most commonly cause uterine dehiscence. Rupture of the uterus can be confined to the dehiscence or the end of the scar with an intact overlying serosa and may not communicate with the peritoneal cavity and the hemodynamic sequelae may be absent or minimal. However a full thickness rupture may cause severe hemodynamic problems because of a massive hemoperitoneum and carry a considerable maternal and fetal mortality. The classic scar rupture is said to occur before rupture, whereas lower uterine rupture tends to occur after labour. US: protruding portion of amniotic sac, anterior abdominal wall defect and hemoperitoneum. Occasionally the intra-abdominal contents may be sucked into the uterine cavity producing a bizarre mass. An intrauterine subchorionic hematoma adjacent to the site of a previous cesarean scar is also said to be suggestive of a uterine rupture.

Ovarian vein thrombosis

This is an unusual post-partum complication and seems to be associated with endometriosis, abortion, PID, and pelvic surgery. It is a potentially life-threatening situation with a risk of pulmonary embolism. US: the thrombosed ovarian vein is seen as a tubular retroperitoneal hypoechoic or hyperechoic structure running from the pelvis to the IVC parallel to the psoas muscle. The ovary may be enlarged and hypoechoic and associated hydronephrosis may be seen on the ipsilateral side due to ureteral compression, although the degree of pelvic dilatation may be difficult to assess in the post-partum patient. Ascites may be present. The thrombus may extend into the IVC, which can be assessed by duplex and color Doppler.

Luteoma of pregnancy

Luteoma of pregnancy is a rare cause of a non-neoplastic ovarian mass that emerges during pregnancy and regresses spontaneously in the immediate post-partum period. It is usually an incidental finding but can be hormone-producing elaborating androgens, producing maternal and fetal hirsutism and virilization. The recognition of this abnormality is important to avoid unnecessary surgical intervention with concomitant maternal and fetal risk. The tumors vary from a few millimeters to over 20 cm in diameter. Sonographically they appear solid with either a single or multiple nodes, and can be unilateral or bilateral. Complex cystic appearance has been described because of hemorrhage. The sonographic appearances are not specific and differentiation from ovarian neoplasms is not possible. But since malignant tumors are rare in pregnancy and luteomas regress spontaneously, masses compatible with luteomas may be observed over a short term in the post-partum period in the appropriate clinical setting.

Retained of products conception

Products of conception may be retained with an abortion or after culmination of a full-term pregnancy, secondary to post-partum hemorrhage or infection. Predisposing causes: succenturiate lobe or placenta accreta, increta or percreta. Uterine atony and focal genital ulceration may be contributory factors. The value of US in the diagnosis of retained products has not been defined. An endometrial thickening >5 mm associated with focal fluid collection has been associated with retained products. A hyperechoic endometrial mass has been shown to have a positive predictive value of 90% for retained products of conception. Doppler US has been shown to demonstrate low-impedance flow three days following delivery irrespective of uterine appearance. Low-impedance flow beyond this period may be associated with endometrial debris and endometrial thickening.

Intrapelvic hematoma

Hematomas should be considered in the differential diagnosis in patients with pelvic pain and fever in the post-partum period. Bladder-flap hematomas following low transverse incisions for cesarean section are seen as solid or complex masses between the uterus and posterior bladder wall. Hematomas anterior to the bladder may occur as a result of disruption of the inferior epigastric artery during caesarean section or traumatic vaginal delivery. These hematomas may be seen as complex or echogenic masses anterior to the bladder or posterior to the rectus sheath.

Inversion of uterus

This is a rare complication of misplaced pressure on the uterine fundus or traction on the cord of non-separated placenta usually in a multiparous woman in whom the uterus dimples and inverts. In severe cases the fundus turns inside out and may herniate through the vagina. This is usually a clinical diagnosis but US may show the in-folding of uterus with a bizarre layered appearance of the uterus. Hydrostatic pressure can be attempted and monitored by sequential sonograms.

Gynecological

Pelvic Inflammatory Disease (PID)

The severity of PID ranges from isolated endometritis to tubo-ovarian abscess and diffuse peritonitis. The clinical presentation can be variable and sometimes non-specific depending upon the degree of pelvic organ involvement and type of infective organism. Sonographic findings are again related to the severity of organ involvement. In early PID the US appearances may be entirely normal. Endometritis may be suspected with fluid in the uterine cavity, uterine enlargement and effacement of the endometrial echo-complex. The appearance of air within the endometrial cavity is further evidence of endometritis although air may be normally present in post-partum women in up to 21% in the first 3 weeks after delivery. Tubo-ovarian abscesses may present with a tubular folded structures. Fluid is common in the cul-de-sac and may be septate. With extension of the inflammatory process to the ovaries and the tubo-ovarian complex the ovaries become ill-defined and can no longer be identified as separate structures. The uterine outline is ill defined. Although the US features are non-specific a fairly confident diagnosis can be made when the clinical presentation is taken into account. In the absence of appropriate history differentiation from endometriosis, pelvic neoplasm, ectopic pregnancy, adnexal torsion and hemorrhagic ovarian cyst may be difficult by sonography alone.

Adnexal torsion

US findings depend on the degree of vascular compromise and the presence of the adnexal mass. US findings of ovarian torsion vary with age. In neonates and young children ovarian masses appear extra-pelvic (abdominal) whereas in pubertal girls the ovarian mass is adnexal. The ovary may appear normal particularly in children but may displace structures such as gestational uterus or the ovary, which may contain a mass, e.g. cyst/cystic teratoma. One of the most consistent findings in ovarian torsion is the increase in volume of the affected ovary to 26–441 ml (normal volume = 7–7.5 ml). The affected enlarged ovary frequently shows multiple cysts peripherally placed, some as large as 2.5 cm in diameter. Other findings include a complex adnexal mass and fluid in the cul-de-sac. Doppler signals can be demonstrated in many twisted ovaries but Doppler US features are not specific and overlap with a number of other gynecological disorders such as PID, ectopic pregnancy, ruptured ovarian cyst and appendicitis.

Hemorrhagic ovarian cyst

Hemorrhage within luteal and follicular cysts are not uncommon. The majority present in patients under the age of 40 years, with a sudden onset of lower abdominal pain. Hemorrhage also occurs in malignant ovarian cysts, most being serous adenomas usually in post-menopausal women. US: features depend upon the stage at which the examination is performed after the onset of hemorrhage. Increased through transmission is present in 90% of the hemorrhagic cysts confirming their background cystic nature. When evaluated within the first few hours most hemorrhagic cysts are hypoechoic although most are heterogeneous. The cysts become increasingly hypoechoic with the passage of time. A fluid-debris level or septate mass may be seen. A solid hyperechoic mass may occur due to the presence of blood clot. In the event of a cyst rupture the cyst may no longer be visible or may be seen as thick-walled irregular mass. Free peritoneal fluid and fluid in the cul-de-sac may be detected in the event of a cyst rupture. An acute hemorrhage may be isoechoic to ovarian stroma and may be associated with an enlarged ovary. Large cysts are less likely to resolve spontaneously.

Massive edema of the ovary

Enlargement of one or both ovaries due to accumulation of edema fluid in the ovarian stroma, which present with an acute or intermittent lower abdominal pain in females aged 6–33 years. Chronic edema of the ovary may cause masculinization. The cause is postulated to be obstruction of ovarian venous, drainage/ lymphatic drainage due to partial or intermittent obstruction. US: solid/multicystic adnexal mass.

Mittelschmerz

Pain prior to or at the time of ovulation said to be related to expansion of the ovarian capsule by pressure from the Graafian follicle. US: may show a sudden decrease in follicular size over minutes to hours as a result of rupture of the mature follicle. Fluid/blood may be demonstrated in the cul-de-sac.

Hepatic subcapsular hematoma

Rare but potentially life-threatening complication of pregnancy, most occur in second or third trimester pregnancy but may occur in the immediate post-partum period associated with a multitude of causes (vide infra). US: crescent-shaped collection of echogenic fluid just beneath the liver capsule, over time the hematoma becomes more hypoechoic and cystic. Septations and echogenic debris may be observed. In case of hepatic capsular rupture the echogenic matter may extend into subphrenic and subhepatic spaces.

HELLP syndrome

HELLP (Hemolysis, Elevated Liver enzymes, Low Platelets) is a syndrome associated with pregnancy with a high maternal mortality (3–24%) and perinatal mortality (8–60%). It occurs in 4–12% of patients with severe preclampsia/eclampsia. The patients usually present with headaches, nausea and vomiting, peripheral edema, epigastric and right upper quadrant pain. US: pleural effusions, ascites, enlarged bright liver (fatty infiltration) with hypoechoic/hyperechoic focal areas within the liver, which represent areas of liver necrosis and subcapsular hepatic hematoma.

Acute fatty liver of pregnancy (AFLP)

An unusual subtype of a fatty liver occurs in association with pregnancy. The incidence of AFLP is 1:10 000 to 1:15 000 deliveries. Typically the patient presents in the third trimester of pregnancy with non-specific symptoms such as nausea and vomiting and abdominal pain. The disease eventually progresses to liver failure coagulopathy, encephalopathy, and renal failure. Early diagnosis is essential as AFLP has a high maternal and fetal mortality (85%). With early diagnosis mortality has been reduced to <20% in the past 20 years. US: fatty hepatomegaly (bright liver) which may be associated with splenomegaly and ascites.

Acute ureteral obstruction of pregnancy

'Physiological' hydronephrosis and hydroureters occur in 90–95% of asymptomatic women in the third-trimester. Mild ureteral dilatation can appear as early as the first trimester. Right-sided dilatation predominates in 80–90% of pregnant women. The ureteral dilatation seldom occurs below the pelvic brim. The pelvic/ureteral dilatation resolves within a few days but more often over a few weeks and in most females the urinary tract returns to normal within 6 weeks. In some there is progressive dilatation throughout the pregnancy. Pregnant women presenting with an acute flank pain is a challenging diagnostic problem. In the absence of pyrexia and leukocytosis the differential diagnosis is generally between a calculus-causing obstruction and compression of the ureter by the gravid uterus. In either case treatment is conservative and symptomatic. If pain persist or increases then imaging is required. Interpretation of US may be difficult since most pregnant women in the second half of pregnancy have pelvic/ureteral dilatation. If US demonstrates a normal renal pelvis or only minor dilatation of the renal collecting system obstruction is unlikely. But moderate or severe hydronephrosis on the symptomatic side is suggestive of an obstructing calculus or hydronephrosis of pregnancy. A prominent left hydronephrosis in a patient with a left flank pain is highly suggestive of a ureteric calculus obstruction as 'physiological' hydronephrosis of pregnancy on the left is either absent or mild. Women with ureteral compression from the gravid uterus can usually be managed conservatively by postural drainage, i.e. lateral decubitus or knee-chest position, failing which a ureteral double pigtail catheter or percutaneous placement of a nephrostomy catheter may give relief. The documentation of the presence of ureteral jet bilaterally with color Doppler effectively excludes ureteral obstruction in non-pregnant patients. But in a pregnant patient the finding of a unilateral jet is not a reliable sign of ureteral obstruction and so would not differentiate between obstructive and non-obstructive hydronephrosis during pregnancy. Jets in pregnant women are few in number and often asymmetrical.

Pregnancy pyelonephritis

Bacteriuria, often asymptomatic, is not uncommon in pregnant women (2–7%); of these 20–30% would develop acute pyelonephritis if bacteriuria is not treated promptly. US is the preferred investigation for acute pyelonephritis in the pregnant female, which may reveal calculi, hydronephrosis, perinephric abscess, renal abscess or air within the kidney/renal pelvis. Pregnant patients with pyrexia, flank pain, leukocytosis and pyuria usually have pyelitis or pyelonephritis and respond well to antibiotics. However if symptoms persist and there is underlying hydronephrosis, pyonephrosis should be suspected and only prompt establishment of urinary drainage can save renal function in these cases. US may show hydronephrosis with echogenic fluid content.

Kidney rupture

Spontaneous rupture of the renal pelvis/kidney is a rare complication of hydronephrosis of pregnancy and may occur before or after labour. US: decompressed renal pelvis associated with fluid around the kidney.

Gynecological Causes of Ureteral Obstruction

- Ovarian vein thrombosis
- Endometriosis
- Ovarian remnant syndrome
- PID
- Ectopic pregnancy
- Uterine prolapse
- Hematocolpometra

Pregnancy Associated Causes of Subcapsular Hematoma of the Liver

- Preclampsia/eclampsia mostly seen in multiparous women after 20 weeks
- Acute fatty infiltration
- Abruptio placentae
- DIC
- Acute cholecystitis
- Rupture of the uterus
- Sepsis
- Thrombotic thrombocytopenic purpura
- Hepatocellular carcinoma
- Hemangioma
- Liver abscess
- Possibly the contraceptive pill
- HELLP syndrome

Mimics of Obstetric/Gynecologic Emergencies

- Gastroenteritis
- Diverticulitis
- Appendicitis
- Pyelonephritis
- Renal calculi
- Complications of Crohn's disease

Further Reading

Burke BJ, Washuwich TL (1998) Ureteral jet in normal second and third-trimester pregnancy. *JCU* 26: 423–426.

Chan ADS, Gerscovich EO (1999) Imaging of subcapsular hepatic and renal hematomas in pregnancy complicated by preclampsia and HELLP syndrome. *JCU* 27: 35–40.

Choi JR, Levine D, Finberg H (2000) Luteoma of pregnancy: Sonographic findings in two cases. *J Ultrasound Med* 19: 877–881.

Yaakaji V, Nghiem HV, Winter TC (2000) Sonography of obstetric and gynecological emergencies: Part I. *AJR* 174: 641–549.

Yaakaji V, Nghiem HV, Winter TC (2000) Sonography of obstetric and gynecological emergencies: Part II. *AJR* 174: 651–656.

Index

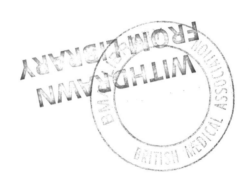